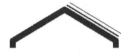

The Middle Falls Time Travel Series

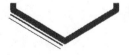

The Unusual Second Life of Thomas Weaver
The Redemption of Michael Hollister
The Death and Life of Dominick Davidner
The Final Life of Nathaniel Moon
The Emancipation of Veronica McAllister
The Changing Lives of Joe Hart
The Vigilante Life of Scott McKenzie
The Reset Life of Rebecca Wright
The Tribulations of Ned Summers
The Empathetic Life of Rebecca Wright
The Successful Life of Jack Rybicki
The Many Short Lives of Charles Waters
The Stubborn Lives of Hart Tanner
The Alternative Life of Aiden Anderson
The Encore Lives of Effie Edenson
The Regretful Life of Richard Bell
The Anxious Lives of Edwin Miller

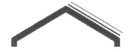

Copyright

The Death and Life of Dominick Davidner

By Shawn Inmon

©·by Shawn Inmon 2017

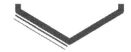

This book or parts thereof may not be reproduced in any form, stored in a retrieval system, or transmitted in any form by any means without prior written permission of the authors, except as provided by United States of America copyright law.

Kindle Edition License Notes This ebook is licensed for your personal enjoyment only. This ebook may not be re-sold or given away to other people. If you would like to share this book with another person, please purchase an additional copy for each person you share it with. Thank you for respecting the author's work. The views expressed in this work are solely those of the author.

Published by Pertime Publishing, 2017

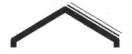

For Dawn

I would search for you for many lifetimes

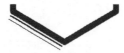

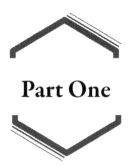

Part One

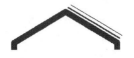

Chapter One
Dimension AG54298-M25735
1999

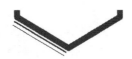

The day Dominick Davidner died, he awoke with a smile on his lips.

"Hey, old girl," Dominick said, laying his hand on Emily's hip. "You're going to be late for class if you keep snoozing."

Without opening her eyes, Emily mumbled, "I'm the teacher. I can't be late, because they can't start without me." She rolled toward him and opened one eye. "And what the heck is this 'old girl' stuff? I am still but a child, taken advantage of by an older man."

"Six months. I am six months older than you. That is not exactly robbing the cradle." He brushed her blonde hair, now with streaks of gray finding their way in, away from her eyes and kissed her. "Happy anniversary, Mrs. Davidner."

"Oh, please. You know I'm diabetic and can't handle this much sugar in the morning." She groaned as she rolled out of bed and slipped her feet into her slippers. "Maybe you were right the first time. I am an old girl."

"Just as beautiful as ever, though."

"Mmmmph," Emily said, shuffling toward the bathroom.

An hour later, coffeed and ready for the day, Dominick kissed her goodbye. "Tonight. Dining. Dancing. Maybe even some of that hootchie kootchie I hear the kids talk about."

"Promises, promises," Emily said.

They got into their cars—hers four years newer than his, but still not new—and headed in opposite directions.

THAT AFTERNOON, DOMINICK sat in the teachers' lounge at Middle Falls High School. "Why don't you take my last period for me, Zack?"

Zack Weaver, the PE teacher and track coach, was in his early forties, but looked younger. He laughed and put his feet up on the table, his hands behind his head. "You know what? I'd love to, but they don't let old jocks like me teach the hard classes. I'm gonna spend sixth period in my office, getting ready to go home. You are suffering from the weariness of being a real teacher." He winked at Dominick. "This is what you get for being an English teacher instead of a track coach. You've got to actually teach the little bastards."

"Ah, I love 'em." He looked sharply at Zack. "Even your twins, who might be just a little too smart for their own good."

Zack shrugged. "Any smarts they got came from Jennifer, not me."

"But," Dominick continued, as though Zack hadn't interrupted, "I'm hoping to get out of here early enough so Emily and I might have a shot at beating the traffic in Portland."

"Driving all the way to the big city, huh? Nice."

"Ten years, man. Ten years she's put up with me. She deserves more than one nice night out in the city, but on two teachers' salaries, that's all she's getting."

Dominick glanced at the clock in the teacher's lounge.

2:03. I better hustle.

"Gotta run," he said over his shoulder to Zack.

He slipped out of the teacher's lounge and quick-stepped down the hall to his classroom. He closed the door behind him just as the bell rang.

He smiled at the small class. There were only six students in sixth period AP English. There weren't many kids interested in taking the toughest advanced English class.

"Let's continue our discussion of *Lord of the Flies*. Now, where were we?" He flipped his own copy open to the bookmark. "Ah. Right. We were talking about how both Ralph and Simon are perceived as 'good' characters, but—"

CRACK! CRACK! CRACK!

Three sharp reports came from down the hall.

Dominick stopped, held his hand up, and listened.

Two more reports. Louder. Closer.

Gunshots?

School shootings in Jonesboro, Arkansas; Springfield, Oregon; and Columbine High School, had put safety issues at the front of many teachers' minds, but there was no security in place yet at Middle Falls High, and no locks on the classroom doors.

Dominick ran to the light switch and turned the overheads off.

We went over this at the safety meeting. Pull the shades. Turn the lights off. Keep the students in the room.

He turned to the class. Adrenaline pulsed through him, but he kept his voice calm.

"Not sure what's happening, but let's take proper precautions. Doug, pull the shades down. Let's make it as dark as possible in here.

There might be more shooters outside. Make it hard for them to see in.

Everyone else, let's get you into the closet."

He ran to the locked closet at the back and fumbled for his keys. His hands were sweaty and the adrenaline made his hands shake. He got the closet open and hustled the five girls inside. He saw that Doug was pulling the last shade down.

"Hustle up, Doug. Let's see if we can all fit in the closet."

The classroom door burst open.

Gerald Fleischer, a boy Dominick had taught in an English class the year before, strode in. Greasy hair fell over his forehead. He wore a long, olive drab trench coat and he had two pistols in his hand, held horizontal to the ground, like tough guys do in movies. They looked too big for his small hands, and they wavered.

Dominick glanced to his right. Doug had frozen in place, a deer caught in headlights. The closet door was still open.

Michelle Landry made a small "Eek!" of terror, but reached out and slammed the closet door shut.

The color ran out of Doug's face as he stared at the two shaking guns There was nowhere to run to, nowhere to hide.

Dominick willed his legs to take one tentative step toward Gerald Fleischer.

Gerald swung both guns to bear on Dominick.

"Oh, hey, Mr. D.," Gerald giggled. His laugh hinted at insanity. "I'm not gonna kill you. But," he waggled the gun in his left hand at Doug, "this guy's gotta go."

Dominick launched himself.

Time slowed.

Dominick had run track in high school. That had been more than twenty years ago.

As Dominick dove toward Gerald, arms outstretched, the shooter's head turned, eyes wide. He jumped in surprise, which caused him to pull both triggers simultaneously. The bullet from the gun in his left hand ripped through the blinds, shattering the window. The bullet from the right slammed into Dominick's throat.

Dominick jerked in a half-circle, a crimson spray arcing across the room.

Dominick fell, sprawling face-down on the cool linoleum. A pool of blood spread toward his eye, but he couldn't move, couldn't even blink.

As consciousness faded, his last words were, "I'm so sorry, Em ..."

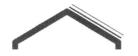

Chapter Two
1968
Dimension AG54298-M85678

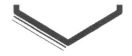

Dominick opened his eyes with a gasp and stared into the wide brown eyes of a dark-haired cherub sitting on his chest. His hand flew to his throat, but there was no blood, no pain.

The cherub's lower lip quivered. "Bubby okay?" she asked.

Bubby? What the hell? No one ever called me Bubby, except Connie. He closed his eyes, hard, and tried to focus.

Wait.

He shook his head slightly, focused on the chubby-cheeked face in front of him. "Connie?"

The worried look fled and the tiny angel rewarded Dominick with a smile and a full body hug.

Dominick disentangled himself from her arms, sat up, and looked around. He was in a small, hot living room. Brown paneling covered the walls. A picture of Jesus knocking on a garden door hung on the wall. A small side table had a framed picture of a smiling couple sitting on the steps of a church.

"No way," he said quietly. "Our house in Emeryville? This place doesn't even exist anymore. It got torn down for condos."

He sat on the floor of a small living room. A couch, stripped of cushions, was behind him. The cushions were scattered like stepping stones across the floor to the kitchen.

"Bubby, lava."

"Lava?" Dominick asked.

The small girl nodded seriously. "Burning."

A memory snapped into place.

Lava. The floor is lava. That's really Connie. But how? She's living in San Jose with her husband. Her kids are teenagers.

"It's okay, Connie. Game's over for now." *Wait. What is going on? Why does my voice sound like that? I sound like a little kid!*

Dominick stood up and caught a reflection of himself in the window. He was tiny, with a mop of curls and spindly arms. The room spun and he passed out, smacking his head against the thinly carpeted floor.

An unknown time later, Dominick opened his eyes, staring into the eyes of the Cherub who was, impossibly, Connie, his baby sister, now truly a baby again. She looked worried, a frown finding unlikely purchase on her unlined face.

"Bubby okay? Why you fall down?"

"I don't know, Squig." *That's right, isn't it? When she was little, we called her Squiggle Butt because of the way she crawled. She got pretty tired of that by the time she was a teenager.*

Dominick stood up to his full height, which wasn't tall at all. "It's okay, Squig. Bubby's okay."

But I'm not. I'm not okay at all. Where the heck, when *the heck am I? I'm forty-one years old. Today's my tenth anniversary. I'm taking Emily to Portland tonight to celebrate.* The thought, the distance, chilled him. *Shit. Emily!*

Dominick turned and ran down the still-familiar hall. School pictures hung the length of the wall. He dashed into the small bathroom on the right. He didn't even have time to flip the light on before he was on his knees. He threw up what looked like macaroni and cheese.

I don't even like macaroni and cheese. He spit a long ribbon into the bowl. *Maybe this is why.*

Shaking, he unrolled some toilet paper, wiped his mouth and flushed. He turned to the sink and had to stand on his tiptoes to scoop some water to rinse his mouth.

He sat down heavily on the toilet.

C'mon, think. I was in my classroom, that little asshole Gerald came in and shot me. I tried to stand, but couldn't. I closed my eyes and opened them here. Based on how little both Connie and I are, that would mean this is sometime in the sixties. But, that's totally impossible. Right?

He sat there for a long time, waiting to see what was next, but what was next was that nothing changed. He heard a crash from the living room.

He ran out and found Connie in tears, the remains of a table lamp broken at her feet,

"Sorry, Bubby, sorry ..." she dissolved again into tears.

"It's okay, Squig. It's okay. Here," he said, repositioning the couch cushions. "Do you want a glass of milk?"

Sensing she wasn't in trouble for breaking the lamp, the tears dried up. She nodded.

"Okay, jump up to the table and I'll get you a glass of milk."

He was barely tall enough to open the upper cupboard, where the plastic glasses for the kids sat on the bottom shelf. He grabbed one, poured half a glass of milk and sat it on the table.

"Connie, where's Mom or Dad?"

She shrugged her shoulders.

"Is anybody else here?"

She looked at him with her head cocked, as though these were things he should already know. She shook her head.

He heard the crunch of tires over gravel in the driveway outside. He ran to the kitchen window and looked outside. Joe Davidner's beat up '55 Plymouth Savoy wagon rolled into the yard. It rattled and wheezed, then finally went quiet.

A tall man with a hairline moving the wrong direction stepped out of the car. He set a black lunchbox on top of the car, then reached back in to retrieve something. Dominick's heart skipped a beat. He ran to the front door, banging his hip against the kitchen counter. He didn't care. He threw the front door open, jumped down the three front steps, and threw himself into his father's arms.

"Dad!, Dad!"

"What's all this, then?" Joe Davidner said. He reached down and picked Dominick up with one arm, light as a feather. "Everything okay, Nicky?"

Dominick didn't want to pull his face away from his father's neck. He breathed in the smell of sweat, tobacco, and grease. Finally, he did, and reached out and held his father's stubbled face in his child's hands. Tears sprang to his eyes.

"I missed you, Dad."

"Did you now? Since this morning? I think something must be broken in the house if you're acting like this." Joe's words were serious, but his eyes laughed. He sat Dominick down on the top step.

"Well, yeah, we kind of broke a lamp. I'm sorry, Dad."

"You'll need to tell your mom you're sorry. She's in charge of lamps. Was it you, or Hurricane Squig?"

"Well, it was both of us. We were playing with the couch cushions and when we put them back, we kind of knocked off the lamp."

"'We,' huh? That little girl doesn't know how lucky she is to have two big brothers covering for her. Speaking of which, where's your brother?"

"Sam?"

"Yes, Sam, unless you're mother's had another son I don't know about, God forbid." Joe made a quick sign of the cross—spectacles, testicles, wallet, and watch—to ward off that thought.

"I don't know. I haven't seen him."

"If that boy was ever where he was supposed to be, it would be a miracle."

Unselfconsciously, Dominick reached up and took his father's hand as they walked inside. As soon as Joe sat his lunch bucket on the counter, Connie jumped down from the table and ran to him. He scooped her up in his arms.

Dominick wandered into the living room, picked up the remaining couch cushion and replaced it.

Somehow, this is all real, then, isn't it? I'm really here. But how? More importantly, why?

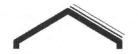

Chapter Three
Universal Life Center

Carrie bent over her pyxis, her brows knit in concentration and concern. "Bertellia?"

"Bertellia is away. I am covering her duties." A disembodied voice, aloof and irritated, came from over her left shoulder.

"Oh! Oh, I didn't know. Who are you?"

"I am her supervisor, Margenta. I am quite busy. What do you want?"

"I just have a question ..."

"I assumed as much. Why else would you have called for me?"

Are there no pleasant people in this part of the universe?

"One of my charges has been recycled, and I don't understand why."

A woman appeared beside her desk. She had iron gray hair pulled up into a bun. Her thin lips were curled back as though she smelled something unpleasant. She reached a long finger out, flicked Carrie's pyxis casually, then smoothed it to a halt. She bent slightly, peered down the end of her nose and watched.

"All is in order. Nothing to be concerned about."

"I don't understand. He was started over. He didn't kill himself. He should have been able to go on."

Margenta sighed impatiently. "Didn't he?" She tipped the Pyxis slightly so the picture grew. The scene showed a young boy, holding two guns. "Listen. This boy says he is not going to harm him. He took action, exposing himself unnecessarily to danger. He died. He was recycled to a starting point."

"That's not right. It's not ..." Carrie was going to say, 'fair,' but she knew better. Her Training Manual had told her time and again that the more she believed in injustice, the longer the journey ahead of her was. She wasn't enjoying eternity, particularly.

"Are you the arbiter of what is right in the universe? Why do you believe that the only people who are started over are those who end their lives prematurely?"

Carrie paused, choosing her words carefully. "Because that's all I've seen. All my charges are people who voluntarily end their life. The same was true for me. Each time I ended my life, I started over in the same place. When I was killed, I ended up here."

"Perspective is everything. A person who lives their whole life in a deep ditch many miles long, but very narrow, might draw the conclusion that the world is only a few feet wide. That doesn't make it so. There are so many things that exist that you haven't seen that you literally cannot imagine them."

Her lip curled a bit. "Bertellia has been far too soft on you. There is no reason for you to care about what happens to this person or why. Like all of us, he is perfect and cannot be truly harmed. Only his circumstances, the appearance of danger, are present." She fixed Carrie with a severe look. "You have one job: feed the Machine. You see the tiniest piece of the universe and yet believe you know what is best more than the Machine that created it." Margenta shook her head. "Sheer hubris."

She was gone.

Chapter Four

Dominick slipped away to look at the rest of the house. The layout was still familiar, even though he hadn't seen it in three decades.

This old house really only had two bedrooms, but I remember when Connie was born, Dad converted the laundry room into a kind-of bedroom for her. So, Mom and Dad's room is there, Connie's is tucked in over there, and there's the room Sam and I shared.

He pushed that door open and stepped into the gloom. A heavy blanket was draped over the one window in the room, blocking out almost all the light. Dominick wrinkled his nose. It smelled of little boy funk—sweaty socks, dirty underwear, and small stashes of hidden food, forgotten about and gone over.

"We were such pigs," Dominick muttered. "Poor Mom. Hopefully, she lost all sense of smell by the time we were teenagers."

Dirty clothes were tossed randomly across the frame of an old wooden bunk bed. A pile of comic books spilled off the bottom bunk and onto the floor. Dominick quietly shut the door behind him. He sat on the bottom bunk—*his* bunk, he knew—and tried to think.

I just hugged my father, who's been dead for twenty years. I held my baby sister, who really is a baby, not the soccer mom *I saw a few months ago. I'm sure Sam will come roaring in any minute. Mom too, I'll bet. It's quite the trip down memory lane.*

Dominick held his head in his hands, an oddly adult gesture in a child so small.

But. Emily. His throat grew thick. *Somewhere, you are all alone, mourning me. Or, are you here, too? Are you a little girl back in Sheboygan again? You always told me that my impulsiveness would get me in trouble, didn't you, Em? When you're right, you're right.*

He closed his eyes, reached out with his mind, his heart, and tried to find her. There was nothing but the silence of the room and the far off ruckus of Connie running through the house.

Em, you were my missing piece. I knew it the first time I saw you. But I was twenty-eight years old on that happy day. What am I now? Maybe eight or nine? I don't think I can wait twenty more years to see you. I guess I don't have any choice, unless I can come up with a plan.

Dominick sat on the bed as the minutes ticked by, waiting for a plan to materialize. None did.

Am I just going crazy? I can touch and feel the things in this room. I know they are real. That other life with Emily, I can't see or feel. It's all just a memory now. So, which of these realities is real? Or, is this maybe Purgatory? What the heck did they teach me about Limbo in Catechism? Am I stuck here until someone prays my way out? Will anyone other than Emily be praying for me? I should have lit more candles.

With a sigh, he slipped off the bunk and walked into the living room just as Laura, his mother, came in the front door. Dominick ran to her and wrapped her in a hug.

"Oof," she said, and raised her eyebrows in the direction of Joe, who was sitting in his recliner with the newspaper in front of him and a beer beside him.

"No idea," Joe said with a shrug. "He did the same thing to me. Check and see if he has a fever."

"Psh, there's nothing wrong with a boy hugging his mother. You've got to let me go, though, Nicky, or I'll never get dinner started."

Dominick turned his face up to her, arms still around her waist. "But you just got home. Aren't you tired?"

"Maybe he does have a fever," Laura said, a faint smile crossing her lips.

Sam, who Dominick hadn't even noticed, snuck up behind him and slapped him across the back of the head. "Let her make dinner. I'm hungry!"

"Sam! Don't hit your brother," Laura said. Sam instinctively ducked, but it was too late. Laura slapped him on the back of the head, but not hard. A warning shot across the bow. "Don't worry, I won't let you starve. If Nicky will let me go, I can put my purse down and get dinner started."

Dominick let go and looked around. Laura was already in the kitchen, hamburger frying on the stove. Joe was relaxing in his chair, the paper open to the sports page. Connie was running up and down the hallway, singing a nonsense song about frogs. Sam had turned on the television—black and white, Dominick noted—and was sitting on the floor in front of it, absorbed in an episode of *Gilligan's Island*.

This is your life, Dominick Davidner.

Dominick sat on the couch and pretended to watch the show on the television, but his mind was elsewhen.

Twenty minutes later, he was pulled from his reveries by his mom saying, "It's on the table. Come and get it before Sam eats it all."

Sure enough, Sam was already at the table, ready to dig in to his plate, but wisely waiting for the rest of the family to arrive.

Joe scooped Connie up as she blitzkrieged past him, carried her to the table and sat her on the Funk and Wagnall dictionary that sat on the chair next to Laura's spot. The plates were already loaded—Wonder bread with a hamburger patty and canned chili spread over it. More slices of Wonder bread sat in the middle of the table, next to the butter. A tall glass of milk sat by everyone's plate but Joe's. He had brought his Budweiser from the living room.

Everyone but Dominick dropped their head and reached their hand out. When he was slow to react, Connie looked up and whispered, "Bubby!" With a start, Dominick took his father and little sister's hand.

"Bless us, oh Lord, in these thy gifts," Joe intoned, "which we are about to receive from thy bounty. Through Christ, our Lord, Amen."

Before the last syllable was out of Joe's mouth, Sam had crossed himself, and in one smooth motion that spoke of long years of practice, picked up his fork and scooped a huge mouthful of chili burger into his mouth. While everyone else was still straightening out their napkins, Sam had already loaded a second forkful and it was lined up like an airplane waiting for a landing clearance.

Dominick glanced at his mother to see if she would rebuke Sam for bolting his food, but she ignored him. Apparently, that battle had already been lost, and she felt no need to put forth a renewed effort. Birds had to fly, bees had to buzz, and Sam had to eat.

Dominick turned his attention back to Sam. He wasn't really fat, just soft. Fat was still a few years off for him, or at least it had been in the life Dominick had just left. Where the rest of the Davidners had dark, curly hair, somehow Sam had straight, sandy hair and freckles. "An Irishman in the woodpile," his father liked to joke.

Dominick cut through the chili, hamburger and bread with his fork and butter knife. He looked up to see everyone staring at him. Sam's mouth hung slightly ajar, showing an appalling mixture of milk and chili.

"What?" Dominick asked.

No one answered, but instead went back to eating. A moment later, Joe said, "What is this, Nicky? High tea with her majesty?"

Dominick looked down and realized he had cut his food into neat little squares, arranging them just so on his plate.

"What's wrong with you, spaz?" Sam asked, helpfully.

"Nothing," Dominick said, pushing the pieces into more of a mess.

Joe reached over and slapped the back of Sam's head without even looking up from his food.

It's a wonder we didn't grow up concussed.

Sam didn't even seem to notice. He pushed himself halfway out of his chair and glanced hopefully at the stove. "Any more, Ma?"

Laura glanced at Joe, who shook his head slightly.

"Sure, honey, there's one more patty and a little more chili over there. Here, give me your plate and I'll fix it for you."

Without a word, Sam handed over his plate and buttered a piece of bread to eat while he waited.

Life is so different. Emily and I split chores and housekeeping 50-50. Here, Dad works all day, comes home, and he's done. Mom works all day, then comes home to cook and do the dishes. What are the odds she's got a load of laundry to do before she goes to bed?

When dinner was done, Joe picked up Connie, said, "C'mon, Squig, let's get you a bath and ready for bed."

Guess I shouldn't judge him too harshly. He loved us. He was a product of his time. What would somebody from 2030 have thought about the way we lived in 1999? They might think we were full of crap, too.

On the way out of the kitchen, Dominick passed by Sam, who hip-checked him into the refrigerator, rattling the jars inside.

"Hey, hey, boys! No roughhousing!"

"Sorry, Ma. He slipped."

Laura gave him *the look*, then turned back to clearing the dishes.

Sam turned to strut away, victor once again, as he had been a thousand times before.

Dominick shot out his foot and caught Sam in mid-stride. Sam tumbled forward, fell, and smashed face-first into the cupboard under the sink. The crash reverberated through the tiny house. The cupboard door swung open violently and hung askew on one hinge. Stunned, Sam sat up, blood dribbling from his nose.

"Dominick!" His mother shrieked.

"What in holy hell is going on out there? It sounds like the whole house is coming down!" Joe shouted from the bathroom.

"You're dead," Sam mumbled, pinching his fingers over his bloody nose. He scrambled to his feet and reached for Dominick, murder in his eyes.

Laura grabbed Sam, tilted his head back, and pushed dirty paper towels against his bleeding nostrils.

He beat me up just about every day, growing up. If I'm going to be here for a while, I've got to draw a line in the sand. He's bigger than me, but thirty years of extra living' and a couple of years' worth of judo lessons at the Y's has got to be worth something, right?

"Dominick Sylvester Davidner! You apologize to your brother right now."

I'm sorry you were a crappy older brother? That'll never pass.

Dominick put the most sincere expression he was capable of on his face, and said, "Sorry, Sam. I didn't mean to trip you."

"Baloney, you didn't!"

Laura turned her attention back to Sam's injured nose, and Dominick let the sincerity slip away. He smiled innocently at Sam, then winked.

Sam's mouth fell open again. It was dawning on him that something had changed. This wasn't the same little brother he'd been pushing around for as long as he could remember.

Dominick walked to his father's chair, picked up the newspaper and looked at the date on the front page: August 2, 1966. *I just turned nine years old then. Guess I missed my birthday party. If I'm here, I guess Emily is probably in Wisconsin. So, how does a nine year old kid get from California to the upper Midwest with no money and no hope of getting any? And, if I were to somehow get there, what do I say? "Hi, Emily, it's me—your future husband. Don't you recognize me?" An easy way to get a one way ticket to a rubber room, even for a kid.*

Dominick eased into his father's easy chair. It was several degrees beyond *broken in*, with silver duct tape holding the seat together in three places. He opened the paper to the front page.

His father, standing over him, cleared his throat loudly. Dominick looked up and raised his eyebrows, as if to say, "Yes?"

"I knew it would come to this, but I didn't know it would come so soon. You're challenging me for leadership of the house? So be it. What will it be? Tickle fight? Pillows?"

Dominick's face was a mask of confusion.

"Don't play dumb, Nicky. You know the rules. Only Dad sits in Dad's chair when Dad is in the house."

"Oh! Oh, gosh, I forgot about that!" Dominick jumped down quickly, red touching his cheeks.

Joe ruffled Dominick's hair, said, "All right, then, I'll let you live to grow a bit more before you challenge me." He sat down, wrapped an arm around Dominick's waist and pulled him onto his lap. "Gave your brother a bloody nose, did you?" he asked quietly.

Dominick nodded.

"I understand. I grew up with two older brothers, and your Uncle Tony and Uncle Frank weren't always easy on me." Joe pulled his hair away on one side and leaned forward slightly. "You see that scar there?"

Dominick leaned forward, then reached a tentative finger out to touch it.

"We were climbing a small cliff in the woods behind our house. Since I was the youngest, I was the slowest one up. Your Uncle Frank dropped a chunk of granite the size of your fist down on my head."

"That bastard."

"Nicky!" Joe exploded. "Language!" He couldn't hide the laughter in his voice, though. "I'm only telling you so you know I understand. It's hard being the littlest. I know Samuel can be a little tough on you, like my brothers were on me. You can't slam his face into a cupboard, though. Got it?"

"Got it, Dad." *I love you, Dad. You were a good man, and I've missed you.*

"Good. For now, then, we'll call that your one free shot to even the books, so no punishment. You can help me fix the cupboard tomorrow, when I get home from work, though. Deal?"

"Deal." Dominick said, placing his tiny hand inside his father's rough grip.

"No more bloody noses for your brother, though, or you won't get off so easy next time, *capiche*?"

Dominick nodded solemnly. "Got it, Dad.'" He laid his head against his father's chest, listening to the strong heartbeat, loving him.

That night, when Sam climbed the small ladder to the top bunk, his right foot shot out toward Dominick's head. Dominick was ready, though, and the kick missed him by half a foot.

"I meant to miss you, twerp. Just a warning."

Dominick waited until Sam was creaking above him, then said, "Hey, Sam? You remember Uncle Frank and Uncle Tony, don't you?"

"Well, duh," Sam said.

"You remember they were both older than Dad, right?"

"I guess. So what?"

"Tonight, Dad told me that when he got to be about my age, he started fighting back every time they picked on him. By the time he'd bloodied their noses a few times, they figured out they should find someone else to pick on. Dad told me I could do the same thing to you."

"Nuh-uh."

"Yep, he did. Ask him for yourself. I think he feels sorry for me, because he was smaller, too. Doesn't matter to me, ask him for yourself."

"I will, you know."

By the uncertainty in Sam's voice, Dominick could tell he wouldn't.

Dominick smiled and snuggled down into his pillow.

I wonder if I'll still be here in the morning?

Chapter Five

While Dominick slept, he dreamed. A swirling kaleidoscope of images, colors, and emotions that coalesced into one face. Emily. She stood on a rise in the middle of a small field. Dominick walked toward her, but the more he walked, the farther away she appeared. The field gave way to mud, and Dominick's feet stuck more and more with each step. Frustrated, he stopped, reached his hands out toward her and shouted her name.

Dominick's eyes fluttered open. A hand was gently shaking his shoulder.

Emily? He focused instead on his mother's face. *Oh. Guess I'm still here.*

"Nicky, I know it's Sam's day to watch Connie, but he's such a bear to wake up in the morning. Do you mind getting up and sitting with her until he gets up? Then you can go play with your friends."

"Sure, Mom," Dominick said, throwing the covers back and setting his feet on the floor. "I've got her."

"Thanks, sweetie. She's bright-eyed and bushy-tailed, having her Cheerios. Don't lay back down, now," she said, hurrying out the bedroom door. "I'm already late for work."

Dominick stood up on tiptoes and watched Sam sleeping. "You were already making allowances for him, weren't you, Mom?"

At 10:30, Sam finally wandered into the living room, hair askew, dressed only in his Fruit of the Looms.

"Mom asked me to watch Connie while you got your beauty sleep. She knew you needed it more than I did."

Sam brushed past him without acknowledging his presence, poured himself a bowl of cereal, and sat with his back to the living room to eat.

"I'm gonna go outside. Mom said I could leave as soon as you were awake."

Without looking, Sam raised his hand over his head and waved, middle finger extended.

Dominick kneeled down, looked Connie in the eye. "Try not to break anything, okay, Squig?"

"'K, Bubby."

Dominick kissed the top of her head. "You sure were a cute toddler."

He went outside into the already-hot August morning.

Dominick walked around his yard. It wasn't much—a falling down picket fence, patchy brown grass, and a one-car garage behind the house.

Typical for Emeryville in the sixties, I guess. You'd never know this place would be a high-tech haven in another thirty years. In the sixties, it was meat packing plants, manufacturing, and blue-collar jobs. Pixar isn't even a glimmer in anyone's eye yet. It was an okay place to grow up, I guess, but it always felt like we had just missed out on living somewhere cool. A few miles west, Haight-Ashbury and the counterculture will be kicking off. A few miles north, it's Berkley, and the University. Of course, a few miles more to the south, it's Oakland, so it could be worse.

Dominick walked to the small garage and pushed the side door open. It was dark inside, but the light switch turned on a single bare bulb, dangling from a cord. The heavy air smelled of dirt, oil, and gasoline, mixed together into a heady potpourri.

Almost all the interior space of the garage was taken up by a black 1942 Dodge Town sedan. Dominick smiled to himself. *Dad* said he was fixing up this old Dodge for twenty years. I think eventually, he finally admitted he was never going to do anything with it, and sold it, so someone else could dream about fixing it up.*

Dominick stood back and looked at the Dodge appraisingly. It had no tires, and sat on concrete blocks. The windshield was cracked, and a thick coat of grime covered the whole vehicle. He pushed his nose against the dusty driver's door window and looked inside. It was slightly better inside than out. The upholstery had a few tears, but everything else looked worn but functional.

I'll bet we could get it up and running in a few weekends, if we tried. I'm a better than average mechanic, and Dad was always kind of a genius with holding stuff together with chewing gum and bailing twine.

He walked outside, squinting into the bright sunshine and saw two boys about his age walking through the gate. One was a black boy, tall and thin with a good start on an afro. The other was short and slight, with straight dark hair. *Oh, crap. They look familiar. I know them, I know them.*

"Hey, Dom!" the young black boy said.

What's his name? In a flash of insight, it snapped into Dominick's brain.

"Hey, Wardell, what's up?"

Wardell and ... and ... Vinny! Yes, Vinny! My two best friends when we lived here. I remember that we spent a lot of time together, but what did we actually do all day?

"Wanna head down to the bakery?" Vinny asked. "It's Wednesday, so Mr. Miller might be there by himself. Mrs. Miller is so tight she squeaks when she walks, but he's nice. He might flip us a cookie or some doughnut holes."

"Sure," Dominick said. *I have no idea what he's talking about or where the bakery is, but yeah, sure, let's go. Is this my life, then? Hanging out with little kids all the time? I might go a little crazy. Still, it would be cool to see what the town looked like back then. Er, now. Whatever.*

The three boys turned right out of the yard and followed a meandering path along a cracked sidewalk. Everything seemed to be of interest to them—a weird bug crawling up a fence, a stray dog, a hubcap jammed into the V of a tree.

I guess this is what we did.

It took them forty-five minutes to walk ten blocks. Vinny picked up a stick and rattled it along the picket fences as they passed, making a satisfying thunk-thunk-thunk sound. Wardell and Vinny talked the whole time and didn't appear to notice that Dominick wasn't joining in.

I feel lost. They obviously know me, and trust me, but I can barely place them. This whole situation would almost be easier if nobody knew who I was.

They had left the neighborhood of small houses behind, and approached the edge of the business district, when they saw three other boys approach from the opposite direction.

"Oh, shit," Wardell said. "Billy Stitts. I hate that guy."

Wardell, Vinny, and Dominick moved closer to the brick wall of the dry cleaners they were passing by, trying to blend in and give most of the sidewalk to Billy and the other two boys. Instead of passing by, though, the three older boys stopped.

"Hey, look who it is, moron number one, two, and three," Billy Stitts said, cracking himself up.

The two other boys, Brian Halloran and Dick Woods, laughed too. "You're funny, Billy," Brian said.

Vinny tried to push by and get around the corner to freedom, but Dick, who was built like a future offensive lineman, blocked his path. The three older boys had been wandering aimlessly, but had found three bugs they could torture with a magnifying glass.

"Wait a minute," Billy said, zeroing in on Dominick. "I know you. You're Sam Davidner's little brother, aren't you?"

Dominick gazed back at Billy. "Yep."

"I hate that prick. Last week, he called my sister a whore."

Way to go, Sam. Ever the diplomat.

"I want to give your brother a message from me." Quick as a shot, Billy's fist shot out and connected with the soft flesh between Dominick's shoulder and collarbone.

"Ow!" Dominick said, and without thinking, pushed back against the bigger boy, who stumbled backwards. Billy tripped over the curb and nearly fell, but caught his balance at the last minute.

"Uh oh," Wardell said, under his breath.

Billy smiled, a mean, petty smile that showed small, yellow teeth. He lifted his right fist above his shoulder like he was about to take off in flight, and bull rushed Dominick.

Dominick stood his ground until the last minute, then shifted his weight to the left, caught Billy's right wrist with his right hand and used it to catapult Billy toward the brick wall. As Billy flew past, Dominick thrust his left hand out, lightning-quick, and pushed hard against Billy's elbow. Three sounds followed in rapid succession: the snap of Billy's elbow as it broke, the pop of his shoulder as it dislocated, and the thud of his face as it slammed into the brick wall.

Snap, crackle, splat.

Thank you, Judo Night at the "Y."

The four other boys stood looking down at Billy with mouths agape.

A banshee wail came from Billy, crumpled on the sidewalk, writhing in pain, trying to find a non-existent way to hold his right arm that didn't result in waves of agony.

"Oh, man," Wardell said. "You crushed him."

"I didn't mean to. I didn't have time to think about it. It just happened."

Mr. Chen, who owned the dry cleaners, pushed open the door to his shop to see what the screaming was all about. "Hey, you kids! What are you doing? You are scaring off my customers! Get away!"

Dick Wood pointed down at Billy, then at Dominick. "I think he killed him!"

Billy's high-pitched scream continued non-stop.

"C'mon, Dom, let's get out of here," Vinny said.

"I think I need to wait here, explain what happened."

"Like hell you do," Vinny said, grabbing Dominick by the arm and pulling him in the direction they had come. "Let's go!"

The three boys ran, Wardell in the lead, Vinny dragging Dominick by the arm.

"Holy crap, Dom! Where did you learn how to do that?" Wardell yelled over his shoulder as he ran.

"I saw somebody do that on TV," Dominick answered.

"I'm watching the wrong shows!"

Chapter Six

Wardell and Vinny walked with Dominick back to his house. They made the trip in just a few minutes this time—no time for bugs or hubcaps after what they had just seen. At the gate to Dominick's house, the other boys split off for their own houses for lunch, still buzzing about the destruction of Billy Stitts. The legend, only minutes old, was already growing.

Dominick walked into the house. Sam was lying on the couch, watching a movie. From the ruckus he heard, Dominick guessed that Connie was jumping on the bed in her room.

Should I tell Sam that his big mouth just about got me beat up? Or, that I might be in trouble for breaking Billy's arm? Probably not. Nothing to be gained.

Dominick sat down in his father's chair and tried to focus on the movie.

It was a long afternoon. Dominick tried to eat something, but his stomach was upset. The more time that passed since his confrontation with Billy, the worse he felt about it.

I should have just let him punch me. What would have been the worst thing to happen? Maybe I get a black eye or a bloody nose? So what?

Five o'clock brought a replay of the day before. Joe rolled into the driveway first, carried his lunchbox in and swept up Connie in a hug, then grabbed a Budweiser and sat down in his chair. A few minutes later, Laura came in, changed out of her work clothes, and started bustling around the kitchen making dinner.

Dominick sat on the couch, holding an *Incredible Hulk* comic book in front of him, and stewing. *What's best to do? Just hunker down and hope the whole thing passes? Broach the subject now? If so, with whom? Mom? Dad?*

They had just sat down to a dinner of what his mother called hamburger hash—crumbled hamburger mixed with boiled potatoes and onion—when there was a knock on the front door.

All conversation, scraping of silverware against plates, Connie's non-stop chatter, even chewing, stopped. A knock on the door during a Davidner dinner was a rare event.

Joe raised his hand, said, "Don't everyone get up at once. I'll get it."

Dominick could hear his father opening the front door, and muffled conversation, but he couldn't hear anything more than that. After just a few moments, he heard his father say, "Laura, I think you need to come here."

Laura dabbed at her mouth with a paper towel, then disappeared around the corner. Sam continued to shovel hamburger hash in, oblivious to any drama that might be about to play out. Connie, on the other hand, seemed very interested in where everyone had gone.

"Where Mama, Bubby?"

"She'll be right back. Here, eat some of this potato," Dominick said, prodding a piece with his fork. "It's cool now."

Dominick's stomach did flip flops. *I know this is about me. Who is it, the cops? Did I make this whole trip back here just to end up in Juvenile Detention?*

A moment later, Laura came back into the kitchen. She looked as though she might be seeing her youngest son for the first time. She wiped bits of potato and hamburger off Connie's face and picked her up, settling her on her hip. She turned to face Dominick.

She stared at him for a long moment before she said, "Billy Stitts' father is here. He's on his way home from the hospital. He says you broke Billy's arm today."

That was enough to catch Sam's attention. "No way! That's awesome," Sam said with a chortle.

Laura looked sharply at Sam. "No, Sam, it's not awesome. They think he might have done permanent damage to his arm. It's not awesome at all. Finish your dinner. Dominick, come with me."

Dominick nodded miserably and followed his mother into the living room. His father was standing next to a man Dominick had never seen before. Sitting on the Naugahyde couch, looking even worse than Dominick felt, was Billy Stitts. His right arm was in a cast from his hand all the way to his shoulder. The cast was bent at a forty-five degree angle at the elbow, so it could fit in the sling he wore. He didn't have black eyes yet, but the redness, puffiness, and butterfly bandage across his nose spoke of their imminent arrival.

Ned Stitts was a big man, taller than Joe, and outweighed him by forty pounds. He was dressed in jeans, work boots, and a well-worn chambray work shirt rolled up at the sleeves. The clothes and boots had both seen better days, as was true of Ned himself. He eyed Dominick suspiciously, turned to Joe and said, "No, it can't be this one. Don't you have another son?"

Joe nodded and over his shoulder, shouted, "Sam!"

A scene like this was one of the few things that could draw Sam away from an unfinished plate of food. He came around the corner, still chewing. "Yeah?"

Mr. Stitts looked appraisingly at Sam, then nodded, as though he found him more acceptable. He nodded his head at Sam and said, "It's gotta be that one, right, Bill? The big one?"

Billy looked away, staring at the painting of Jesus. He shook his head slightly.

"Really? The scrawny one? What the hell, son?"

Billy continued to look anywhere other than at his father.

"Dominick," Joe said, "Mr. Stitts says that you did all this to his son. You want to tell me what happened?"

I really wish now that I'd told you this earlier.

Dominick sucked in a deep breath and said, "Wardell, Vinny and I were walking around downtown this morning. We ran into Billy and two of his friends. Billy said that Sam had called his sister a whore last week –"

"Samuel!" Laura said, more upset at the use of that word in her house than she had been by the battered boy on her couch.

Sam flushed and tried to melt back into the kitchen.

"I'll deal with you next, young man. Dominick, I never want to hear that word in my house again, understood?"

Dominick nodded. "Anyway, Billy said that he wanted me to take a message back to Sam. Then he punched me. It hurt, and it kind of made me mad, so I pushed him away. He was off balance, and he almost fell down. Then, I think he got mad, because he ran at me. I jumped out of the way, and he ran into the wall."

Okay, not one hundred percent truthful, but close enough to give me plausible deniability, I hope.

Mr. Stitts waved a piece of paper in front of him. "What are you going to do about this, Davidner? The hospital bill came to over $350!"

Welcome to 1966. I can only imagine what that would cost in 1999.

Joe took the paper and looked it over. He was silent for a long minute before he said, "You're in the meat packing union, so you've got insurance through them, right?"

Stitts nodded.

Joe continued, "This is August. You've got a wife and three boys, I'm willing to bet you've met your deductible already, haven't you?"

Again, Stitts nodded.

"So, that covers 80% of it. That leaves, what, Laura?"

"Seventy dollars."

"Right, seventy dollars. It sounds to me like both our kids made a mistake, and maybe even your kid started it. Just because yours got the worst of it doesn't give us any obligation—"

"Now wait a minute—"

Joe held his hand up. "But, we'll still do the right thing. Laura, go get the checkbook and write Mr. Stitts a check for thirty-five dollars. I think that's more than fair."

Dominick watched Stitts face work. After a few seconds, he said, "Fine."

I think Dad missed his calling. He should have been a union rep with those kind of skills.

"Good, then. That's settled. Do you want a beer?"

"The sun hasn't risen on the day Ned Stitts turns down a beer."

"Good enough." Joe went into the kitchen.

For a moment, it was just Dominick and father and son Stitts. Ned narrowed his eyes, obviously unable to figure out how this little wisp of a boy had beaten his beefy son badly enough to send him to the hospital. "So, you boys are all square now, right?"

"Yes, sir," Dominick said.

"Billy?"

Billy looked like he would rather be anywhere else than sitting on the couch of the smaller boy who broke his arm. Still, he managed a nod.

"Not good enough, son. I need to hear you say it."

"We're square."

"If I hear of you starting something with either of the Davidner boys, I'll break your other arm myself."

Joe came back into the living room and handed the check and a Budweiser to Ned.

Ned tucked the check into his shirt pocket, cracked the beer and made a small salute with it before draining a quarter of it in one long gulp. He wiped his lips with the sleeve of his shirt and said, "Well, we've gotta take off. The old lady's out in the car."

Dominick nearly laughed at the absurdity of that image—Ned and Billy Stitts inside the house, Ned with a beer in his hand, while Mrs. Stitts sat quietly in the car, waiting—but he managed to squelch it in time.

He tried to slip quietly back to his bedroom, but Joe caught his eye, shook his head, and said, "Come here, Dominick."

Joe sat in his chair, grabbed Dominick by the arms and stood him straight in front of him. This would not be a "sit in Dad's lap" conversation.

"This is a serious, Dominick. You really hurt that boy."

Dominick nodded, but didn't say anything.

"You've been awfully different the last few days. I don't know what's going on, but it's going to stop. I guess I shouldn't have let you off so easy when you bloodied Sam's nose. This is what comes from sparing the rod."

You talk tough, Dad, but I don't remember you ever whipping us, no matter how much we deserved it.

"How much is your allowance?"

"Oh, crap. How much *is* my allowance?"

"Don't act dumb with me, Nicky. Your allowance is fifty cents per week. If I take the whole thirty dollars out of your allowance, you won't have any gum or candy for a year, which is what you probably deserve. But, here's what we're going to do: no allowance for you from now until Christmas, plus you're going to put an extra hour in on chores, helping your mother every Saturday before you go play with your friends. Understand?"

"Yes, Dad. I'm sorry. It all just happened really fast."

"That's the way it is with life, Nicky. It all happens fast."

AFTER THE EXCITEMENT of the dinner hour, things settled down at the Davidner residence. No one but Sam felt like finishing dinner, so Laura gathered the leftovers into Tupperware for Joe's lunch the next day. Joe got Connie tucked into bed and everyone settled into the living room—Sam on the floor in front of the television, Joe in his chair, and Laura and Dominick on the sofa.

Laura patted the cushion beside her. "Come here, Nicky, sit next to me."

The Scolding, Part Two? No fair. Dad already gave me my talking to.

Dominick scooted over and Laura pulled him close. She stroked his curly hair. "Nicky, Nicky. You've always been my gentle boy. What's going on with you?"

You'd never believe me if I told you, Mom.

"Two fights in two days with much bigger boys and you come out unscathed. It's so unlike you."

Dominick didn't answer, but just buried his face against his mother's side.

"After church on Sunday, I've arranged for Father Wilkins to come by the house and talk to us."

"Us?"

"Well, your father, me, and you."

"But mostly me."

"Us," Laura said firmly.

Chapter Seven

Sunday was the one day each week that the Davidners were all up and around at the same time. No laying slugabed on the Sabbath. The family didn't overdress for church, but the kids were bathed, their hair was as combed as it ever could be, and the five of them were in the car headed to Mass by 7:30. It was a constant question of whether to get out of bed early to make the 8:00 AM mass and have the rest of the day for chores and the Raiders, or to get a bit more sleep and go to the 10 AM mass.

Joe and Laura sat up front in the Plymouth with Connie between them and the two boys in the back. When he climbed in, Dominick automatically pulled the seatbelt out, which had been stuffed deep into the crack at the back of the seat, and clicked it into place. Sam just looked at him and shook his head, as if to say, *my brother the weirdo.*

"You won't think I'm odd if Dad rear ends somebody and you go head first out the windshield and into the back of a semi."

"I might be dead, but I'll still think you're a weirdo."

"Fair point."

It was another warm morning, and the sun shone against the brick exterior of St. Augustine. Inside, the church was cool, with that slightly damp, but not unpleasant, smell that seemed to exist only in churches. Everyone, even Connie, dipped their fingers into the Holy Water and made the sign of the cross before genuflecting at the edge of the pew and taking a seat. Once in the pew, Laura lowered the kneeler and the whole family kneeled for a moment of silent prayer and reflection.

Dominick clasped his hands in front of him, lowered his head, and prayed fervently. *God, I am so confused. I have always done my best to follow You and Your Word. Now, I feel so lost. Everything I once thought I knew, seems false. Please help me find some clarity, some understanding. What lesson am I supposed to learn? I am your servant. I only need to know how to serve. Please let me hear Your Voice.*

The church bell rang above their head, calling people in to worship, and Dominick felt his throat tighten and tears leak through his closed eyes.

Those bells get me every time.

He felt his mother's warm hand on his back and when he turned his head, he saw she was smiling at him gently.

Dominick looked around. Tall ceilings, graceful arched stained glass windows, paintings of the Stations of the Cross hung between them. At the front, the altar stood tall, draped in white cloth with a purple sash. A seven-foot-tall Christ hung on the cross on the wall behind. To the right of the altar was a statue of a blue robed Mary, Mother of God, arm outstretched, offering peace to the congregation.

When Mass started, Dominick's swell of emotions drained away. The priest stood with his back to the congregation and conducted the service in Latin.

What the heck? I don't remember this. How many of us speak Latin, anyway? How are we supposed to keep up? How do we share in this and experience the sacred? It's all ceremony and no connection with the congregation.

Inevitably, Connie began to fidget impatiently, and Laura searched through her purse to find something to entertain her, finally settling on a compact mirror, followed in short order by a roll of butterscotch LifeSavers.

Soon enough, Joe and Laura had gone to the front for Communion, and shortly thereafter, the service was over. The tall doors of the church were thrown open and warm summer sunlight poured in. The Davidners emerged, blinking, into that sunlight, the troubles of the previous day forgotten for the moment.

Once home, everyone took off their church clothes and hung them back up for the following Sunday. Sam threw on a t-shirt, ball cap and jeans, and was out the door in a flash. Dominick did his best to follow his brother's lead, but he was collared by his mother before he could get to the front door.

"No running off, Nicky. Father will be here soon, and I don't want to have to hunt all over the neighborhood for you."

FATHER WILKINS ARRIVED just in time for lunch, which was a bean soup that Laura had made with a hambone from earlier in the week. Like magic, Sam reappeared just as the table was being set.

Nature's great mysteries—the swallows returning to Capistrano and Sam returning when food hits the table.

Father Wilkins said the blessing, then the adults chatted about the weather, the upcoming bake sale, and the health of a number of parishioners. The priest had changed out of his robes, of course, but his black pants and shirt and backward priest's collar still conveyed the message of who was the moral authority in the room. He was a short, stout man with white hair and a stern visage that transformed when he smiled, which he did often.

This is all just stalling. The main event is coming up: Priest vs. Boy. Who will win?

When the soup bowls were empty, Laura suggested they move into the living room for coffee.

Soon, Sam had once again disappeared, Connie was playing as quietly as she ever did, and the adults had their beverages. Joe had traded his normal after-lunch beer for coffee as well. Joe and Laura lit cigarettes and Father Wilkins fished about for his pipe and tobacco.

I wonder if priests think the world is a better place, since everyone is on their best behavior around them, or if they know we're all just sinners that put a temporary hold on it in their presence?

"So, Dominick, your mother tells me you've been having a little difficulty this week."

"Father, why do you say the mass in Latin? Wouldn't it be better in English, so we could understand everything that's being said?"

Father Wilkins sat back in his chair a bit, eyebrows raised. He smiled indulgently. "Well, son, that is the way Peter said the first Mass, so it is the way we have done it for a very long time. There are changes afoot in the Church, but most of those changes have not reached us here in Emeryville yet, so we still do things the way we've always done them. Now—"

"When I die, will I go to Heaven?"

"Nicky, it's not polite to interrupt people when they are speaking, especially Father," Laura said.

"No, no, it's all right, Laura. It's only natural to have questions like this. Answering them is my job. Dominick, we all have an assurance of Heaven if we are faithful to God and keep his Commandments."

Dominick nodded. "I was pretty sure that's what you would say, but it didn't happen for me."

"I'm sorry?" Father Wilkins said, certain he had misheard.

"I died, and when I opened my eyes, I was back here, not in Heaven. I'm just trying to figure out why that happened. I've been asking God, but haven't heard anything back yet. At first, I thought maybe this is Purgatory, but now I don't think so. I think I'm just having to live my life over again, and I'm trying to figure out what I'm doing here, what I'm supposed to be accomplishing."

This rush of words quieted the room, so the only sound was Connie singing *Twinkle Twinkle Little Star* to her stuffed bear.

The adults exchanged glances. Father Wilkins took the lead. "Dominick, are you saying you had a dream like this?"

Dominick let the mask of being a young boy slip away, "There's nothing, really, in any of our theology that would explain this, is there, Father? Catholics don't believe in reincarnation, and that's not exactly what this is, anyway, is it? This is more like I just got dropped back into my life at some random point to do it all over again." Dominick took a deep breath in, held it for a long moment, then let it hiss out. "This is getting us nowhere. I didn't really think you had some secret answers, but I had to check. Okay, then. So, what did you want to ask me, Father?"

Dominick was quickly pushed outside to play. Whatever conversation the priest and parents had planned evaporated when Dominick revealed exactly what his situation was.

Probably not the best idea, but it felt like I had been keeping a secret, ever since I got here. If you can't tell your parents and your priest the truth, who can you tell?

He walked along the side of the house and saw Sam's old bicycle leaning against the fence. Much of the red paint was missing—rusted or just scraped away from many falls—but when Dominick pulled it loose from the grass that was growing around it, everything still seemed to function. He pushed it out through the front gate and tried to jump up. It was a struggle, because it was too tall for him. Eventually, he managed, though, and a moment later, he was pumping the pedals, and whizzing through his old neighborhood, leaving all his troubles far behind.

Chapter Eight

Carrie feathered her pyxis to a stop and looked at the scene in front of her. Dominick Davidner sat on a wooden pew in a church, surrounded by his family. At the front of the church, a priest was chanting a prayer.

A wave of nostalgia swept over Carrie and she let herself be carried along with it. She thought of the tiny church in Middle Falls that she had attended with her mother and father. The same church she had spent nights with Thomas Weaver. The same church she had been murdered in.

I miss those times when I thought I knew what waited after death. I was completely wrong, but I felt like I knew anyway, and in a way, that was as good as knowing. Now, the more I learn, the more I know, the dumber I feel.

She turned to the woman who sat at the desk next to her. "Maruna? Do you ever wish you were still back on Earth, and didn't know all this?"

Maruna, who appeared to be about the same age as Carrie, turned in her seat. Her long black hair was pulled up into a careless fall, her skin was fair, and perfect. She shook her head. "Why would I? It's better to know some small amount with certainty, than embrace a false idea."

"Yes, but I was certain then, too. I proselytized. I tried to live my life as an example to others."

"Mmm-hmmm," Maruna said, and returned to her own pyxis.

"It can be so lonely here, sometimes."
Maruna was not listening.

Chapter Nine

Dominick rode until his legs ached and hunger overcame him.
A bowl of bean soup only goes so far.
I guess I've done it now. I have no idea what's next. Was the Catholic Church doing exorcisms in 1966, or did they wait until the seventies, when The Exorcist *came out? No idea. I wish there was a way I could just get away and not burden my parents like this. They've got enough on their plates just making ends meet. They don't need to worry about having an insane child, too. For all I know that's what I am—insane. I mean, crazy people don't know they're crazy, do they?*

It was almost dinnertime when Dominick pushed Sam's bicycle back into the yard. The kitchen window was open, and he could hear his mother singing softly to herself—an old song he didn't recognize.

What am I walking into here? The Pope Patrol, ready to gather me up and haul me away? Or, worse, a strong talking-to from Mom and Dad.

Dominick pushed into the living room and found Connie sitting on Joe's lap, fast asleep.

She only has two speeds. A hundred miles an hour, or out cold.

Joe put a finger to his lips, and Dominick nodded acknowledgement.

In the kitchen, his mother was just taking a roast out of the oven, a rare treat for a family that survived on hamburger in all its variations. She signaled Dominick to come into the kitchen.

She took him in her arms and held him tight. Before she let him go, she laid a hand against his forehead.

Now I know I've messed things up. I've given Sam a bloody nose, broken Billy's arm, and completely freaked out Father Wilkins, but everyone's still good to me. They must be ready to ship me off to the loony bin. I wonder if Dad's union insurance will cover a long stay in the straightjacket hotel.

A few minutes later, they gathered around the dining room table. They all held hands and Joe said grace.

There wasn't any conversation. No one, not even Sam, seemed to know what to say with a child at the table that might have wandered off the path of sanity. Finally, Dominick said, "Hey, Dad? What are you going to do with that old Dodge out in the garage?"

Joe lit up, happy to be on more familiar ground. "I'll get to it soon enough. It could be a fine machine, just needs a bit of attention."

"Do we need a lot of parts to get it up and running?"

Joe thought for a minute, chewing his roast slowly. "No, not really. I'd need to get a couple of tires patched, and I've drained all the fluids out of her. I'd probably need to rebuild the carburetor, but that's not too much work. Why?"

"I was thinking it would be fun to help you."

Joe stared at his youngest son levelly. Dominick could almost read his thoughts: *He's never showed an interest in cars before. Why now? Is this more of whatever's wrong with him?*

"Sure, Nicky. I was always hoping you boys would be interested in working on it with me. How about you, Sam? Want to help, too?"

Sam shrugged.

Joe leaned over toward Dominick. "I'll tell you what. I'll take the tires that need patching to work with me tomorrow, and I'll stop on the way home and get them done. We can jack it up and put them on tomorrow night after dinner. We can take a look at what else needs to be done, too. Maybe we can all take a Sunday drive in it after church this weekend."

"That would be great, Dad."

Everyone tucked into their Sunday dinner, pleased to have something to think about other than what was wrong with Dominick.

JOE WAS AS GOOD AS his word. He brought two patched tires home on Monday night and he and Dominick pumped them full of air. They soon discovered that the two tires Joe thought were fine also needed a patch or two, though, which put them off another night.

After getting all four tires on, Joe took the carburetor apart and laid it on his cluttered workbench. He pulled a carburetor rebuild kit down from the top shelf and blew half an inch of dust off it.

"Had this sitting here for years now. Guess I was just waiting for you to give me a push, Nicky. I think I'm getting fat and lazy." He patted his midsection, where there wasn't an ounce of fat, then took another chaw of Copenhagen out of the tin he always carried in his back pocket.

It's that stuff that's going to kill you, Dad, not getting fat and lazy. How can I tell you without worrying you more?

"Dad," Dominick said. "You know that stuff's bad for you, right?"

"What, snus?"

"Yeah, it causes cancer too, just like smoking cigarettes."

"Ah, Nicky, they haven't proved that. I think it's just a scare tactic."

Dominick shook his head vehemently.

"No, Dad, it's not. It's real. I love you. I don't want you to die."

Joe turned toward the workbench. "That's sweet, Nicky. I don't want to die, either, and leave your mother with all the bills. I'll think about it, okay?"

Dominick watched his father take the carburetor apart and carefully clean each part with a special cleaner, then set them out to dry.

I worked for three years as a mechanic, but there's something so satisfying about watching someone else who knows what they are doing work on a car.

"We're getting there, boyo."

They spent a pleasant evening listening to Johnny Cash, Charlie Pride and Hank Williams on the tiny radio and working on the car.

LATE SATURDAY AFTERNOON, Joe charged the battery, put a gallon of gas and a few quarts of oil into the car and rolled it out of the garage. It took a few attempts and some cussing under Joe's breath, but eventually, the old Dodge rattled to life. Laura, Connie, Sam, and Dominick stood to the side and applauded.

"Well, it might not be ready for a cross country road trip, but I think it'll make it out of the city limits. We'll take her for a spin tomorrow."

Everyone else went into the house, but Dominick stayed behind, got a bucket and a sponge and did his best to give it a wash. Even standing on the door frame, he couldn't reach the middle of the roof, and the middle of the hood evaded him until he climbed up on it, but when he was done, it looked better than it had before he started.

It's been an odd week. Everyone's acting like I never said anything to Father Wilkins. I guess that's how families get through things like this. Pretend like it never happened and hope it doesn't happen again. What else are you going to do?

At church the next day, Father Wilkins greeted the family on the way out the door. "May the Lord be with you," he said as they passed. Dominick thought that he gave him a bit of a fish eye, though.

At home, Laura put a picnic basket together with sandwiches, chips, and a potato salad she had made the night before and they piled into the Dodge. They held their breath when it took Joe took a minute to get it started, and again when it died just as he was pulling out of the driveway.

Joe said, "Goddamn it," then caught Laura's disapproving look. "I'll go to confession next week, okay, hon?" then jumped out, raised the hood, and tinkered for minute. When he started it again, it ran smoother. He turned left out of their neighborhood and pulled into the Shell station just a few blocks away. He gave the attendant two singles. Dominick leaned forward and saw that pushed the gas gauge up past half a tank.

Joe worked his way to Highway 123, then paused.

He turned to the family. "Whose turn is it?"

"Mine!" Sam said.

"Mmmm, I don't think so, Sam," Joe said. "I'm almost sure it is little Connie's turn. Don't you think so?"

"Yes!" Connie said, nodding emphatically. She looked to her left, then her right. After several seconds of deliberation, she pointed left, as regally as Cleopatra ever could have.

"Left it is, then," Joe said, turning the wheel.

It was another hot August day, so everyone rolled the windows down and let the breeze swirl through the car as they drove. After half an hour, they turned off the highway toward Alvarado Park. The park didn't have much in the way of playground equipment—no swings or merry-go-round—but it was a nice change of pace from the city, with lots of hiking trails to explore.

Laura laid out the picnic lunch while Joe laid down with his arm over his eyes and fell asleep. Dominick played tag with Connie, and Sam even joined in for a while. When lunch was laid out, everyone sat around the checked tablecloth to eat their sandwiches and drank their warm cherry Kool-Aid. Laura surprised everyone with a treat for dessert—a Twinkie for everyone.

For a time, Dominick managed to forget his troubles and be a forty-one year old kid again. It was a break from all the worrying and wondering, but it was not to last.

Chapter Ten

It was Dominick's turn to watch Connie again the next day, so he spent most of that Monday playing with her at the tiny park down the street from their house.

On Tuesday, he was up early, ate breakfast and got out the front door before his mom could ask him to watch Connie until Sam hauled himself out of bed.

He walked along the side of the house and opened the side door to the garage, letting the morning sunlight pour into the dusty darkness inside. He looked at the nail by the door, hoping to see the Dodge's ignition key hanging there, but no such luck.

I know it's too soon to be able to take off for good. I don't have any money, other than what's in that little piggy bank I spotted on the dresser in the bedroom, and there's no way an eight year old kid can make it on their own, even if they are forty-one on the inside. Still. I want to fire the old girl up, take her for a spin around the block. No harm can come of that. Then, when the time comes, I'll know she's ready.

He poked through half a dozen rusty Folgers coffee cans, but was rewarded with nothing more than dozens of different bolts, screws, and nails.

I can't believe he takes the key to this old car with him to work? Who's going to break into our garage and steal this old hunk of junk? Other than possibly me, of course.

Dominick walked out of the garage just in time to see his mother pull out of the driveway on the way to work. He snuck into the house through the back door and into his parents' room. He checked the table beside Joe's side of the bed, but it was bare, apart from the small lamp and a half-filled ashtray. He checked the small drawer in the table on both sides of the bed, but came up empty. Finally, he crept into the bathroom, where the hamper was.

When he picked up his father's jeans, he heard a slight jingle, but it was only a few nickels, pennies, and dimes—no keys.

Okay. Gonna have to do this the hard way. I can hotwire the thing. It's easy on these old rigs. I'll just have to put it all back together before Dad gets home and he'll be none the wiser.

He went out the back door again, then into the garage and pulled the door shut behind him. He grabbed a flashlight, a roll of electrical tape, and a pocket knife off the workbench and lay on his back on the driver's side.

There are some advantages to only being four feet tall.

He pulled the plastic cover behind the steering column off, then pulled the bundle of wires down. He separated out what looked to him like the battery, ignition, and starter wires and gave them a little tug to separate them.

Don't want to cut them. That's too obvious, and Dad's too sharp. He'll know something's up.

Dominick carefully cut a small notch into each of the wires, then connected the battery and ignition wires. The dashboard lit up. He lightly touched the starter wire to the first two and the starter tried to turn over. He reached over his shoulder and gave it a little gas and the engine fired up.

Yes! I knew I could do it. I love these old cars.

He took a small piece of the tape and wrapped the battery and ignition wires.

Sweat ran down his face and he wiped it away with one hand. He hopped out of the car, ran outside the garage and looked around to see if the sound of the Dodge starting had attracted any unwanted attention. The only sounds were the car idling in the garage and Mr. Bratski's lawnmower across the street.

Dominick lifted the garage door up. There was a moment of panic, when he thought he might not be tall enough or strong enough to get the door up all the way so he could drive the car out. Standing on his tiptoes and shoving with all his might, the door finally swung up.

He squinted up at the door. *Now how in the heck am I going to get that back down? I guess I'll burn that bridge when I get to it.*

He climbed back inside the Dodge and put his hands on the steering wheel. If he extended his neck as far as he could, he could just barely see over the dashboard. If he did that, though, his feet couldn't reach the gas and brake.

I guess I should just be happy it's an automatic. I'd never be able to handle the clutch, too.

Dominick scooted his butt as far forward as he could and fished around for the brake with his foot. He found he could touch the brake and gas, *or* he could see out the windshield.

Damn. Maybe I should just shut this down and wait another *year or so, until I've grown another few inches.*

The Dodge idled noisily, filling the garage with fumes.

Or, I could just figure it out on the fly. I like that option better. One step closer to freedom.

Dominick pressed the brake and shifted into drive. The car pushed forward a few inches, then he let off the brake and it rolled toward the street.

If Sam looks out the living room window right now, I am totally busted, but if I know him, he's on the couch, looking the other way, watching television.

He gave it just a little gas, doing his best to hold onto the steering wheel, which was huge in his small hands. He hit a bump where he had to cross the sidewalk to get onto the street, and the Dodge rolled to a stop.

Dominick craned his neck left and right to check for traffic, but there were no other cars coming in either direction, so he gave it a little gas. The car rocked against the bump, but didn't go over. He stretched his toes out to give it a little more gas, and his foot slipped, pushing down hard. The car surged forward across the sidewalk and onto the street.

Dominick tried to do two things at once—turn the steering wheel right, and press the brake. He managed to turn the steering wheel, but that threw his balance off and his foot slipped again as it sought the brake.

Oooooh, shit!

Chapter Eleven

"Oh!" Carrie said, adjusting her pyxis. She stopped it completely, then expanded and rewound the scene.

A curly-headed young boy sat behind the wheel of a car that was paused at the end of a driveway. He was obviously too small to drive, but, drive he did. He tried to ease out onto the street, but his foot slipped, and he lost control of the vehicle. It surged across the street. An old man standing in his yard tried to jump out of the way, but was not fast enough.

The car hit him flush, sending his broken body flying up and over the hood, then crashing into the windshield. The young boy finally brought the car to a stop and looked in shock at the body of the man on the spider-webbed windshield. His eyes went so wide, he looked like he might have lost his mind. His mouth formed one elongated word: "Noooooooo!"

Carrie paused her pyxis at that precise moment. She reached into it and plucked a strand of the scene. She backed it up, watching the car careen backwards across the street and up the driveway. She let it play forward again, but the result was the same. She pinched another piece of it away and dropped it into a hole in the floor at her feet.

I know I'm not supposed to interfere. I'm only supposed to watch, and Feed the Machine. That would destroy me, though. Better to do what I feel is right, and end up being fired, or punished, than to just sit here and go crazy. If this is my eternity, I'm going to spend it doing the right thing.

She rewound the scene again, let it play forward.

This time, she nodded to herself, let the pyxis scoop up the emotions—fear, regret, relief—the young boy was feeling.

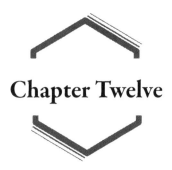

Chapter Twelve

The old Dodge leapt across the street, jumped the curb on the other side of the street and plowed through Mr. Bratski's white picket fence, across the neat front lawn, barely missed Mr. Bratski himself, tore through the rose garden, and slammed into his garden shed.

When the Dodge slammed into it, the shed flew up into the air, bounced off a low hanging branch of an elm tree and came to rest on the hood of the car.

The collision threw Dominick around the car, bashing his head into the steering wheel first, then throwing him clear into the back seat. His temporary tape job on the wires came undone and the engine died.

Mr. Bratski recovered himself enough to run to the car and throw the door open. When he saw that no one was in the front seat, he said, "Is the damn thing running itself?"

Dominick pulled himself up off the floor of the backseat, giving Mr. Bratski a start.

"No sir," Dominick said miserably. "It was me."

Mr. Bratski pulled Dominick from the car roughly by one arm. Dominick steeled himself, believing he was going to beat him severely, and prepared to take it. As it turned out, Mr. Bratski was a nice man, and once the adrenaline rush from being nearly run over had passed, he let go of Dominick and put his hands on his knees, trying to catch his breath.

"Thought I was a goner, for sure, when I saw this old behemoth bearing down on me," he said, then started to laugh. "The Krauts couldn't get me in France, but I almost bought the farm by being run over by a child in an old Dodge." He laughed until he looked up and saw his ruined rose bushes, which had flourished as the result of many hours of babying. The car had cut a vicious swath through them, tearing them, knocking them out of the ground, destroying them.

"Oh, young man, look what you've done here. You've ruined them."

"Yes, sir, I have."

And so much more.

Chapter Thirteen

That day wasn't the worst of Dominick's two lives—getting murdered and taken away from Emily still held the top spot—but it was a good runner-up.

Mr. Bratski had debated with Mrs. Bratski over the right course of action. Which was better—to call the police, or to call Mr. & Mrs. Davidner?

"Who's going to pay for all this?" Mrs. Bratski wondered, wringing her apron in her hands.

"Right," Mr. Bratski had said. "That's why I'm calling his parents. The police aren't going to replace my shed or my beautiful roses."

Just then, Sam came out of the Davidner house, leading Connie by the hand. They both stood, open-mouthed, gazing in wonder and horror at the scene being played out before their eyes. Sam slowly shook his head from side to side, as if he already knew he had been permanently promoted to the best Davidner son.

Slowly, the rest of the neighborhood also came out, and soon it was like an unscheduled block party of concerned neighbors.

Laura Davidner was the first to be able to get away from her job and make it home. She pulled to a too-sudden stop in front of the house, fishtailing slightly, and spraying a bit of gravel.

"Runs in the family," Mrs. Bratski observed.

Laura emerged from her car, with her hand over her mouth in disbelief. She looked both ways, then crossed the street.

"Mr. and Mrs. Bratski, I promise, we'll make this right with you. I don't know what to say."

"To start with," Mr. Bratski replied, "I'd just like to get this car out of my yard, so I can survey the damage."

"Of course, of course," Laura opened the door of the Dodge, climbed in and reached to turn the key. She looked on the floor to see if it had fallen on the floor. "Dominick? Give me the key to the car."

Dominick, standing slightly behind Mrs. Bratski for protection, said, "I can't Mom."

"Of course you can." It was evident to anyone that knew her that Laura was fighting to stay calm, but it was a losing battle.

"I ... I didn't have a key."

"Then how did you...?" She nodded at the destruction in front of her.

"I hotwired it."

"You—you *hotwired* it?" She looked out the open car door at Mr. & Mrs. Bratski. "My eight year old son hotwired our car and drove it into your shed."

"Not to mention my roses," Mr. Bratski offered.

"I'm nine, now, Mom."

Laura leaned forward and rested her forehead on the steering wheel.

Dominick thought she might fall completely apart and dissolve into tears of frustration, but she was made of sterner stuff than that. Laura drew a deep breath, climbed out of the car, and maintaining as much dignity as she could, said, "My husband will be home soon. He will be here to talk to you about the damage and to retrieve the car. I'm so very sorry for what my son has done here. It will not go unpunished."

She took a few steps, grabbed Dominick by the left ear and strode across the street, dragging him in her wake.

TWO HOURS LATER, DOMINICK stood in the hallway, eavesdropping on his father, mother, and Father Wilkins.

His father hadn't spoken to him since he had gotten home. Dominick had watched through the window as his dad had pulled up, spoken to Mr. Bratski, and attempted to start the Dodge. The battery was good. It turned and turned. There was no fire, though, and after several minutes of trying, it became apparent that it wasn't going to start. With Mr. Bratski's help, he pushed the ruined shed off the hood, strapped the Dodge to the station wagon, and pulled it out. It left a new set of massive ruts, right next to the set Dominick had made on the way in.

Being the good neighbor he was, Mr. Bratski helped Joe push the Dodge back into the garage.

With Sam and Connie banished outside to play, the parents and the priest sat in the living room, curtains pulled shut, deciding Dominick's fate.

"Father, what do you advise us to do? This has all happened so fast. A few weeks ago, Dominick was a perfect son," Laura said. "Kind, respectful, thoughtful. Now, all this. Where have we gone wrong?"

Silence filled the room while Father Wilkins filled his pipe from a small pouch, lit it and puffed on it several times. A sweet, woodsy aroma filled the room.

"There are no easy answers, of course, Laura. It's a combination of things. The movies and television shows our children watch these days, the things they are exposed to on the street, the tearing of the fabric of society. It all combines to put a terrible burden on our children."

"What do we do next?" Joe asked. "Lock him in his room until he turns eighteen?"

Father Wilkins chuckled. "Tempting, isn't it? That's an easy thought, when the memory of what they've done is fresh in your mind. That passes with time, though, and it seems a longer term solution is needed here."

Dominick heard a general shuffling, as if someone was shifting in their chair. *Wish I could see what's going on, since it's my life they are deciding.*

"Here's what I have in mind. There's a school up north called Hartfield Academy. I think it's just what Dominick needs right now."

"Hartfield Academy," Laura said. "I'm not familiar. What kind of school is it?"

"It's a military preparatory school."

"Oh!" Laura said, exhaling sharply. "Oh, no. Nicky is so young, so small."

"But the damage he is doing isn't small, is it?" Father Wilkins said, gesturing across the street.

"It's impossible, Father," Joe said. "We're barely making it as it is. Now, fixing the Bratski's yard, it's going to be even tighter. There's nothing left over to send Dominick to a boarding school."

"Of course, of course. I completely understand. You know that I was in the military, don't you? I was an army chaplain for ten years. It was life-changing. It ... well, it made me the man - and the priest - I am today. My commanding officer was Curtis Hartfield III, the same man who runs Hartfield Academy today."

He stopped to suck on the pipe, found it had gone out, and struck another match to relight it.

"I spoke to Commander Hartfield on the phone before I came over today. I called in some old favors, and, well, long story short, if you want it, he's offering Dominick a full scholarship to Hartfield Academy. There would be some paperwork, of course, and we'd have to get a copy of Dominick's records from the school to send along, but he's always gotten good grades, hasn't he?"

Dead silence. Dominick didn't even breathe.

"Yes, but ...," Laura said quietly, then fell silent for a moment. "Well, that's quite a gift, Father."

"I understand, Laura. You're a wonderful mother. You want to protect your son and hold him near. Unfortunately, that's part of what has brought us to this sad state of affairs. A mother's love can only do so much good, before it begins to harm."

Keep going, Father. You're overstepping this time.

"I don't know about that," Joe said. "Laura's the best mother I've ever known. She doesn't smother the boys. We're not going to raise wimps. Until this last week, I've been very proud of both of them."

More shifting of seats.

"But, still ..."

Oh, crap. Really, Dad?

"... I sense the truth in what you are saying, Father. Laura and I will need to talk it over, of course—"

"—Of course," Wilkins interjected.

"—but I think, if Commander Hartfield is really willing to make such a generous offer, we'd be foolish to turn it down. I'm afraid that if we don't, someone else might get really hurt, and then that would be on our conscience."

DOMINICK DID NOT HEAR any of the further conversations between his parents, but three weeks later, he found himself in the family station wagon, on the way to Hartfield Military Academy, just north of Crescent City, California.

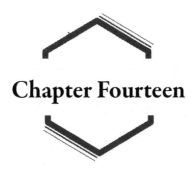

Chapter Fourteen

It was a seven hour drive from Emeryville to the Academy, so the whole family piled into the station wagon while it was still dark. The drive would have been faster, but in 1969, Interstate 5 was still a work in progress, so they stuck to the highways.

Their Sunday drive to the park a few weeks earlier had been carefree and relaxed. This drive had more of the feel of a death march, as everyone was well aware when they left the house that one of them would not be returning.

As they drove north, the weather changed. Temperatures dropped into the upper sixties, threatening clouds filled the sky and gusts of wind buffeted them.

As the miles rolled under the wheels, Dominick stared out the window, lost in thought, deep in self-recriminations. *I think this is best, but man, it hurts. I screwed absolutely everything up. I'm a full-grown man, but something about all this change messed with my head. I wish I'd never thought of us working on the Dodge.*

A little before noon, Laura dug into a paper bag at her feet and fished out bologna and mustard sandwiches wrapped in wax paper and handed them out, along with an apple, and a small bottle of Coke.

Dominick ate his slowly, not completely sure his stomach was going to hold it. In the end, it did.

By mid-afternoon, they rolled through Crescent City, then on to the Academy. They pulled into a Shell station and gassed up.

"Hartfield Academy around here somewhere?" Joe asked.

"Yessir, about four miles further on. There's a big gate on the left hand side. Can't miss it." The white-haired attendant leaned over and glanced in the back seat. "Dropping two off today?"

"Just the younger one, today. Unless they give me a two for one deal and take the other one too."

As they pulled back onto the highway, Sam asked, "You're kidding, right, Dad?"

"Oh, heck," Joe said. "I meant to buy you a sense of humor back at the gas station, but I forgot, Sammy."

"Ha, ha."

A few miles north, there was a break in the trees and a gate with red brick columns and impressive black spikes stood wide open. A small sign read, "Welcome Cadets."

They turned in and drove the long, tree-lined driveway, passing a number of cars going the other direction. The driveway poured them out into a huge open lawn, dominated by a massive gold and black sign that read, *Hartfield Military Academy, where boys become men and men become soldiers.* Behind the sign were two flags—an immense American flag and a smaller, blue and gold one.

Joe and Laura read the sign at the same moment.

"Oh!" Laura said, glancing back at Dominick in the backseat with worried eyes.

"It's all right, Mother," Joe said. "It's going to be fine."

They circled around the long driveway, found a place to park, and piled out, gawking like Iowa tourists in New York City.

Connie had fallen asleep on the last leg of the journey, so Joe pulled her out and laid her head against his shoulder. She slumbered on.

A squat moon-faced boy in a neat uniform stepped forward and greeted the family. "I'm Max. You can call me Max. Welcome to

Hartfield Academy, where we have the best military strategy library west of Washington, D.C."

Joe and Laura exchanged a quick glance, then said together, "Hello, Max."

"You should go into the main building. Registration is in there, and then someone will lead your cadet to his barrack." He looked back and forth between Sam and Dominick. "Both of them?"

Sam took a step back behind his mother, more convinced than ever he was about to be left behind as well.

"No," Joe said. "Just Dominick, here." He put an arm around Dominick's shoulders.

Max focused on Dominick and smiled. "Don't worry. We're nice here. You'll like it." He walked away to greet a new family that had pulled up behind the Davidners.

The main hall had nine-foot-tall doors, which were swung open today. The swirling winds blew some debris inside, but a young cadet manning a broom and a dustpan picked it up and disappeared down a corridor.

Another cadet, dressed in the same immaculate tan uniform, approached and asked, "Registration? It's just down the hall, in the library."

"Thanks," Joe said, and the family trooped in the direction the cadet had pointed.

Inside the library, there was a short line leading up to the desk that normally served as the check out. A man with thinning gray hair was processing a family with a young boy who appeared to be Dominick's age. The boy looked left and right in rapid succession, shuffling his feet.

The man behind the desk handed a packet to the father, then said, "You'll want to keep this, Mr. Summers. It has all the information you will need—how to contact Will if you need to, what our school year schedule is, etc."

Mr. Summers nodded, said, "Thank you," took the packet and turned away.

Joe stepped to the desk and said, "We're the Davidners."

The man picked up a clipboard, ran his finger down it, and said, "Ah, yes. Mr. and Mrs. Davidner and Dominick. I'm Captain Peterson." He turned slightly to face Dominick. "You can call me 'Sir,' or 'Captain,' or 'Captain Peterson.' Understand?"

Dominick nodded. "Yes sir."

"Very good. Now. We've already received Dominick's medical and school records, which are all in order. I'll need you to sign that you understand our discipline policy, and acknowledge that we have the right to fairly discipline your son." He pushed a piece of paper across the desk. "There will be a copy included in the packet I give you." He glanced at Laura's expression and smiled slightly. "Don't worry, Mrs. Davidner. We only have Dominick's best interests at heart."

Joe took the paper, signed it, and pushed it toward Laura. After a moment's hesitation, she signed it as well.

"Are you going to be able to stay for Commander Hartfield's orientation? It's going to be held on the front lawn in," he glanced up at the clock on the wall, "fifty seven minutes."

"I'm afraid not. We've got a long drive back home, and two other children we've got to get ready for their own first day of school."

"Perfectly understandable." Peterson reached under the desk, plucked another packet out, and handed it to Joe. "All the information you need will be in here. There is a phone number, but we recommend that you only use it for emergencies. Especially in the first year, if the cadets hear from home too often, it only increases the loneliness. Of course, Dominick will write home every week, and we encourage you to write him, as well."

Peterson glanced at his left, where a number of older cadets were gathered, talking. "Cadet Pusser?" A stocky blond boy with a bad

THE DEATH AND LIFE OF DOMINICK DAVIDNER

complexion broke away from the others, snapped a salute at Peterson.

"Sir?"

"This is Cadet Davidner. Please escort him to the barracks. Give him a moment to say good-bye to his family."

"Yes, sir," Pusser said, then took three steps backward and stood alert, but at rest.

Captain Peterson smiled at Joe and Laura, then looked past them and said, "Name?"

The Davidners moved outside and walked toward the station wagon. Connie woke up and looked around fuzzily, then laid her head back against Joe's shoulder.

At the car, Sam said, "See ya," and climbed into the back seat, grateful to be on safer ground.

Joe reached out and put his arm around Dominick, pulling him close. He kissed the top of his head and said, "Be good, son. Christmas will be here before you know it."

Laura grabbed Dominick in a fierce hug, whispering, "I love you, Nicky. Be careful, and be good."

Dominick looked up at his mom, who had tears threatening to spill out. He remained dry-eyed and smiled at her. "It's okay, Mom. I'll be fine." He took a step away.

Connie suddenly realized what was happening and reached her two chubby arms out to Dominick, saying, "Bubby, Bubby, Bubby," over and over.

Joe hustled around to the driver's side and slid her into the middle of the front seat. She let out a piercing wail, but Joe quickly started the car and pulled around the great lawn, then disappeared down the long driveway.

Dominick turned to Cadet Pusser and said, "Okay, ready."

The two marched in silence to the First Year's barrack. Pusser opened the door into one long room with a row of bunks on each side and an aisle down the middle. "Grab any bunk that hasn't been taken already. Unpack your belongings into the footlocker, then leave your suitcase on top. It will be stored for you until Christmas. Hustle up, then report out front for orientation. Oh, one more thing. Don't ever be late at Hartfield, and you'll be off to a good start."

Pusser turned on his heel and was gone.

It took Dominick less than a minute to unpack the socks and underwear he had brought and to set his suitcase on the footlocker. He glanced around the room.

Exactly what I would expect. Basic. Utilitarian. Fine with me. Wonder how many of us will be in this class? Doesn't matter, really. Just glad to have a chance to start over, and not have to remember so many things I've forgotten. I don't really want to live the same life over again anyway. That would get boring in a hurry.

Dominick exited the barracks and made his way to the front lawn, where he found a spot with the other First Years. A large man who identified himself as Commander Hartfield came to the podium and spoke for a few minutes about the tradition and brotherhood of Hartfield Academy, followed by a string of instructors who did the same.

Dominick looked around at his classmates. *White bread. Diversity apparently wasn't a big deal in this school in the sixties. Haven't seen a woman or girl on the entire grounds, aside from Moms and sisters.*

Orientation consisted mostly of a long list of rules and regulations, peppered with talk about honor and brotherhood. When it was finished, he went straight back to his barrack and climbed up on his bunk, where he could watch everyone else go about their business. For the most part, each boy stuck to himself. A few made nervous comments or laughed a little, but it was apparent that none of them knew each other. Most appeared to be at least a little scared.

Totally understandable. I would have been, too, if I was really a nine-year-old boy.

The door at the far end of the barracks swung open, and the older boy who had shown Dominick where to unpack strode in. With Dominick, he had been low-key. Now, he appeared to be agitated, almost spoiling for a fight.

""Hello, shit for brains. I am a Tenth Year. I have been assigned as your prefect. I will oversee you for the rest of the year. My name is Lt. Tim Pusser."

Dominick heard a few snickers from various corners of the room. *Typical. Boys will always laugh when they are nervous or scared. Easy way to let off a little steam and fit in.*

Lt. Pusser, his red face showing the ravages of acne even more clearly, focused in on one boy who had laughed at the sound of his name. He took four quick steps toward him and slammed his clipboard into the metal bunk, making a loud BANG that echoed through the room. He spoke in a low, threatening voice, so Dominick couldn't hear what he was saying.

The boy looked like a bug caught on a slide plate. He fidgeted, turned red, and tried to nod and shake his head simultaneously. Eventually the boy dropped to the ground and attempted what looked like a push-up.

Pusser raised his voice, so the whole barrack could hear. "Oh my God! You look like a monkey humping a football, boy! Didn't anyone ever teach you how to do a proper push-up?"

The Lieutenant laid his clipboard down on the bunk, dropped to the ground and pumped out a few army-approved push-ups, then instructed the boy to try again.

I don't think I can just watch this. This school seems like a nice place, but why in the world would they put a guy like this in charge of first year students? I want to just keep my head down and fit in, but I don't know if I can stand by and watch him bully everyone into submission.

Lt. Pusser continued on, loudly reciting the rules of the barracks, including his own personal rules.

I'd say this guy watched Full Metal Jacket *once too often, but that hasn't even been made yet. If this is what being in this school for ten years does to you, I might have to pass.*

While Pusser continued on, Dominick looked around the barrack.

I think I'd like to put a little group together. That'll help. It's a little weird hanging out with nine-year-old kids, but I don't think the teaching staff is going to invite me into their inner circle, so I'll have to make the best I can with what I've got. Don't want to be too eager though. Just have to hang back and watch for an opening. It'll come.

Eventually, Pusser wound down and told them they had thirty minutes before lights out. Dominick hopped lightly down to the ground, next to the boy that would be his bunkmate. He was a small boy with blond hair, already cut in the regulation buzz cut of Hartfield Academy. The rest of the boys wouldn't get theirs until the next day. He stared back at Dominick, but didn't smile or look away. He just stared.

His eyes are haunted. What could give a little boy such an adult expression?

Dominick gave him a non-committal nod and shucked off his clothes, then clambered back up to the top bunk.

Is he something special? He looks more comfortable here than the other kids. I'll keep an eye on him. He might be one to be friends with.

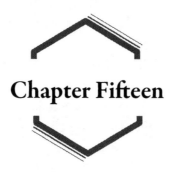

Chapter Fifteen

The next day, reveille was sounded at 6 am, and they had just a few minutes to use the bathroom, brush their teeth, and get ready for breakfast. Everything about the school felt like an assembly line to Dominick. Shuffle from point A to B, sit for an hour, then on to point C.

The first class of the day was English, taught by Mr. Guzman, who Dominick guessed was probably a veteran, as he bore terrible scars on his face, and the left arm of his uniform was neatly ironed and pinned at the shoulder.

After leading the class in the Pledge of Allegiance, Guzman asked a cadet to help pass out the book they would be reading first.

Dominick couldn't help but smile. *The Island of the Blue Dolphin*.

I taught this book my first year in Oakland. I was teaching seventh grade, though, and they're using it in third grade here. That's good. They're tougher here, and at least it's a good story.

Guzman gave them forty minutes to read, then said they would use the last few minutes of the class to discuss the first chapters.

Guzman retreated to his desk, but kept his keen eyes on the class. He watched the pace each student was turning pages, and made notes in a notebook.

Smart teacher. Let everyone read what would be a semi-difficult book for them, and gauge their reading ability without anyone being the wiser.

Dominick opened the book, thinking that he would just pretend to read, but as always when it came to books, he became engrossed in the story and began reading along for real. He made a mental note to slow down, and pause between turning the pages, though. As he did, he glanced to his left and saw that the cadet who was his bunkmate was reading at an exceptionally fast clip. Not quite Evelyn Wood speed reading, but faster than any third grader would have been expected to read.

After only a few minutes, he had finished the first few chapters, closed the book and looked straight ahead. Guzman noticed it immediately.

He'll never buy it. Too fast, kid.

Guzman surprised Dominick by not dismissing him out of hand, but instead walked to the boy and said quietly, "Cadet Hollister. Am I to assume that you have already finished your reading?"

The cadet—Hollister, Dominick now knew—said, "Yes, sir."

Guzman quizzed the boy, and it was obvious that he had indeed read the book.

Either he got lucky and Guzman chose a book he'd already read, or he can read every bit as fast as I can. Interesting.

Through the rest of the class, Dominick continued to read at the same artificially slow pace. *I don't think the class needs two geniuses, and it looks like he's already filling the available slot. I'll just tag along and watch what happens. Still. He's one to keep an eye on.*

In each class, the routine was the same. The teacher gave some work to determine where everyone in the class was, and everyone struggled their way through it, except for Cadet Hollister, who blasted through every assignment.

Either that kid is a certified genius, or ... or, he's like me. Yes! Maybe he's in the same situation I'm in, but he's just decided not to mess around with things, and he's showing them what he can really do.

Dominick thought on that for a few moments, chewing the end of his #2 pencil.

Nah, that's crazy. He's probably just a super smart kid that got dumped here because his parents didn't know how to handle him.

At the end of fifth period—Geography—the cadets were hustled off to get their heads buzzed. Much of America was letting their hair grow into flower power haircuts, but at Hartfield Academy, all cadets wore their hair the same way—high and tight.

Dominick wasn't all that attached to his curly hair, but he saw nervous tears in at least a few boys as they sat in the chair and watched their hair fall onto the growing pile on the floor.

The last period of the day was PE, and Dominick was able to let loose and be himself. Being a forty-one year old man in a nine year old's body didn't give him any special physical advantage, so he could try his best.

Mr. Lawson, who stood out from the rest of the instructors at Hartfield in that he wasn't scarred from war, at least visibly, started them off by running a lap around the quarter mile track. Dominick had run the 440, 880, and mile distances in high school track. He hadn't been talented enough to run for a college team, but he was better than most.

When Mr. Lawson said, "Go!" Dominick took flight, legs and arms pumping. When he hit the exit of the first turn, he looked over his shoulder and saw that no one else was close. He smiled to himself and settled into the rhythm of running—feet pounding a beat on the cinder track, the wind whistling over his now close-cropped hair, his breath burning slightly in his chest.

By the time he sailed across the finish line, no one was close to him. He bent over and put his hands on his knees while he waited for the rest of the boys to cross.

It feels good to run. To be young again. I wasn't out of shape, before. I played racquetball, and Emily and I took a lot of walks, but there's just nothing that can replace the elixir of youth.

Dominick was surprised to see Michael Hollister as one of the last two to cross the finish line.

Guess he's not great at everything.

Dominick went to Michael and said, "Well, that's a relief. I thought you were perfect at everything, but I guess not," then slapped him on the back and ran off to the next exercise, not waiting to see what his reaction would be.

DOMINICK QUICKLY SETTLED into the routine of Hartfield Academy. Each first year prefect had the privilege of naming what mascot the class would be. Pusser was unimpressed with the physical acumen of the boys in Dominick's class, and named them the Turtles. He intended it as an insult, but the boys wore the name like a badge of honor.

The precise schedule and consistent discipline pleased Dominick. Lieutenant Pusser did not. The boy was all bluster and intimidation, leading only by size, strength, and force of will.

At the end of the first week, Dominick and Pusser had their first confrontation. One of the cadets that Dominick had begun to hang out with, Will Summers, had wet his bed. He was humiliated, and tried to cover it up, but Pusser had noticed it on his morning inspection, and pulled Will out of rank.

"Bed wetter, eh? Well, we have a solution to that here at Hartfield Academy. Come here, cadet."

Pusser yanked the blanket back, exposing the damp, yellow stain to the world.

The cadets around Summers faded away.

Pusser pulled the sheet off, compressed it into a ball and turned to Summers. "I said, *Come here,* cadet."

Summers took a half-step toward him, but couldn't muster anything more.

Pusser threw the sheet, hitting him in the face. "You will carry this sheet with you, wherever you go today. I will come looking for you, and if you are not carrying it, then you will carry it with you for a week. Understood?"

Okay, that's it. I can't take this crap any more.

"Lieutenant Pusser, sir, is that really necessary? No one would do this on purpose, and humiliating him doesn't do any good."

Now we'll see how he responds when someone pushes back. He's bigger and stronger than me. I'm sure he can take me out, if he wants to. An image of Billy Stitt flashed across his mind. *If he does, I can't fight back. Better to get a black eye or a split lip than get kicked out of here, too.*

Pusser didn't lash out, though. He walked slowly toward Dominick, smiling broadly. He only stopped when his boots were touching Dominick's. "Davidner, right?"

Dominick nodded into Pusser's chest.

"Where's your bunk, cadet?"

Asshole. He knows very well.

Without looking away, Dominick pointed toward his bunk.

"Top or bottom?"

"Top, sir."

Pusser strode to Dominick's bunk, stripped the green blanket away, pulled the sheet off, crumpled it, and dropped it on the floor. He unzipped his fly and a strong stream of urine splatted onto the sheet. While he was peeing, Pusser looked over his shoulder, made eye contact with Dominick, smiled, and said, "Ahhhh."

He delicately picked the sheet up, walked back to Dominick, and shoved it into his chest hard enough to make him take a step backward. Pusser's urine soaked into his uniform shirt.

"Now. Anybody else got an opinion about this?"

The barrack was silent.

"Good. Now, ladies—"

Pusser was interrupted by motion behind him. Michael Hollister was pulling his own blanket off, then pulling and dropping the sheet on the ground, just like Pusser had done. He peed on the sheet, picked it up, and joined Dominick and Will. He hadn't said a word.

Dominick leaned over and bumped into Hollister's shoulder. He whispered, "I knew you had it in you."

Two other boys—Jimmy Markson and Pete Wemmer followed suit, and then there were five Turtles standing in the middle of the barrack holding urine-soaked sheets.

I think I've found my group.

Chapter Sixteen

That night, the five Turtles who had rebelled against Pusser were sent off to wash their laundry.

Will Summers looked at the other four boys, and said, "This is my fault. Sorry guys."

Dominick laid an arm across his shoulders. "It's no big deal. If we weren't doing this, what would we be doing? Homework? I'd rather be hanging out with you guys than doing that."

"I still feel bad …"

"Could have happened to any of us," Dominick said. "If it wasn't you, it would have been somebody else. I just don't like bullies."

"And that's exactly what Pusser is—a bully," Michael said.

"Yeah, but he's *our* bully, right?" Jimmy Markson asked, with a laugh.

"I guess so," Dominick said. "We're stuck with him, right?"

"Probably," Michael said. "Even if we got rid of him somehow, whoever we get next might be even worse. Pusser's a bully, but he's stupid, so we should be able to manipulate him. Someone else might be smarter."

Dominick looked long and hard at Michael. *Something about that kid. He doesn't speak very often, but when he does, I need to pay attention.*

"The genius speaks," Dominick said. Michael flushed, but Dominick continued, "He's right. If we can just get Pusser to be more of a human being, that's probably better than killing him." He looked around at the other boys with a wink. "Just kidding. He hasn't done anything bad enough for me to kill him. Yet."

OVER THE NEXT FEW WEEKS, the battle between Pusser and the five Turtles of the Yellow Sheet Brigade engaged in a series of running battles. Pusser had the power and the authority, but Dominick, Michael, Will, Jimmy and Pete had ingenuity, daring, and numbers on their side.

The safest thing to do would have been to retreat and wait for the year to pass. Instead, they short-sheeted Pusser's bed, covered the toilet in plastic wrap before he used it, and in general made Pusser's life miserable, mostly without being caught. In return, Pusser gave them an outsized punishment for even the slightest infraction he could find.

The five of them cleaned more toilets, did more deep knee bends, and marched more laps around the track than all the other Turtles combined.

The final battle between Pusser and the five boys came after they took Pusser's underwear from his locker and died it a bright red. That night, when Pusser did his nightly check of the barracks and his own footlocker, his face turned the same color as the newly-dyed underwear.

"Turtles! Attention!"

One moment, there were Turtles scattered around the barrack—on their bunks, sitting playing checkers, on the pot in the latrine—the next, they were lined up at the foot of their bunks, staring straight ahead.

Pusser walked up and down the aisle, pausing for long moments in front of Will Summers, and where Michael and Dominick stood. He held the red underwear up like a flag. "Cadets! Some comedian has taken it upon themselves to destroy my personal property. I have put up with your insubordination in the hopes that you would grow a brain somewhere in those empty heads. I believe I have given you too much credit."

He stopped and stared directly at Pete Wemmer, who stared straight ahead, expressionless.

"Here is what we are going to do. We are going to hold you all at attention until the cadet or cadets who are responsible for this steps forward and takes the punishment they've got coming. I don't care if a fly takes a two-pound shit on your eyelid, you do not move while you are at attention. We will stay like this until someone confesses."

Michael and Dominick didn't move their heads, but gave each other the side-eye, which translated as, *Oh, shit, we may have gone too far this time.*

Lt. Pusser made a show of retrieving a chair and putting it in the middle of the aisle. He straddled it and said, "I've got all night, boys." Pusser's face was calm on the surface, but his neck had turned as red as his underwear.

While being held at attention, none of the boys dared move, but Dominick nonetheless felt their attention on him. Every Turtle knew that when someone challenged Pusser, it was him, or one of the other five that had done it.

Finally, after fifteen minutes of heavy silence in the barrack, he stood up abruptly and said, "I'd rather punish twenty-four innocent boys than let one guilty boy get away with something," He walked back up and down the aisle. "So, I guess that's just what I'm going to do. Here's how it's going to happen. Either the little idiot who ruined my personal belongings will step forward and take their punishment like a man, or every Turtle will be out on that track running laps."

Even while they were held at attention, that brought a groan from the assembled Turtles. As solid as the Hartfield barracks were, they were swaying a bit from the buffeting winds outside, and the temperature had dropped enough to put frost on the grass. No one wanted to leave the warmth of their bunk.

Michael glanced over at Dominick again.

Damn it. I don't want everyone to have to go out in this.

Dominick gave the tiniest shrug imaginable, but it still caught Pusser's eye. He hustled over to stand in front of them.

"Davidner. Hollister. I should have known. It's always you two little shits, isn't it? I'm gonna stick my feet so far up your asses, I can wear you like slippers."

Dominick took a deep breath. *Looks like I'm going to be outside running laps no matter what, so I might as well take it for the team.*

"It's not Michael, it's just me. I thought red was your favorite color, so I was just trying to help you out."

Dominick sensed that Michael was about to throw himself into the soup, too, so he warned him off with a glance and a tiny shake of his head. *No sense in you suffering too.*

"Davidner, you are making me believe in reincarnation, because no one could get this stupid in one lifetime."

You have no idea, Pusser.

"Do you expect me to believe you managed this all on your lonesome? Because I'm not sure you're smart enough to wipe your own ass, let alone do something like this."

Dominick continued to look straight ahead, expressionless.

"Laps, Davidner. Lots and lots of laps. You are ruining my perfect evening by making me go outside in this god-awful storm, so I am going to ruin your night by adding a few more laps. It's colder than a well-digger's butt who's wearing steel underwear out there, so I'm going to get bundled up and stay nice and warm. I want you to change into your T-shirt and shorts."

"Seriously, Lieutenant?" Dominick asked.

You, sir, are an asshole. I understand you want to punish us, but this is too much. What happens if I catch pneumonia and die out there?

Do I wake up in the same place? A different point in my life? That wouldn't be so bad. Maybe if I die again, I'll wake up back in bed with Emily. It's almost worth the chance.

Pusser didn't answer, but strode away and began bundling up in his warmest clothes and overcoat.

Michael whispered, "This is too much, man. We've got to tell him you didn't do this by yourself."

"Sure," Dominick answered. "Then there can be five of us freezing our testicles off out there, instead of just me. Forget about it. I'll do it."

At least, I hope I can do it.

Outside, the freezing rain came down sideways. Dominick was soaked to the skin the moment he stepped from the comfort of the barracks.

The good news is, I should lose all feeling in about five minutes.

He turned to Pusser, barely visible under the layers, and said, "If I start to see a white light, I'm moving toward it, and you'll have to drag my dead carcass back into the barracks and explain what happened to my parents."

"Boohoo, Davidner. I wish you guys would start thinking about this before you do something stupid. Maybe this will help."

Dominick shrugged, then jogged to the edge of the track and started on his first lap. *Running will keep the blood circulating, right? Might as well start picking them up and putting them down.*

On his second lap around, Dominick saw the other Turtles had come outside too. He flashed them a grin as he passed, then concentrated on keeping moving.

As he came around on the third lap, he saw Michael Hollister had dropped his coat and was running in front of him. He caught him by the first corner.

This kid might be a genius, but he can't run for shit. He's gonna slow me down, that's for sure. But still, it's good to find a brother out here.

Dominick slowed his pace, and he and Michael plodded around the track. "Hey, Genius, it's a lot warmer inside. That's where you're supposed to be." Michael just shrugged. The wind, rain, and freezing cold air in their lungs made conversation impossible, so they just kept moving, splashing from one puddle to another. When they came around again, Will, Pete and Jimmy had dropped their coats and were standing, shivering, waiting for them.

Dominick shook his head at them, but couldn't keep from smiling.

Maybe now that he sees that we are all taking responsibility for what we did, he'll let us go back inside.

That was not to be. The Yellow Sheet Brigade pushed on for lap after lap, until whatever joy they had once had at pranking Pusser, whatever unity they had felt at all running together, was drained away. They plodded on, until finally Pusser stood in the middle of the track, held his hands up, and said, "That's it. Head inside. And, if any of you ever touch my stuff again, I will rip off your heads and shit down your necks. Got it?"

The five barely nodded. They headed inside, to the sanctity of the barracks, the warmth of the showers.

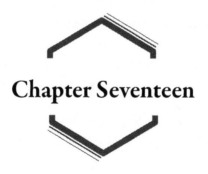

Chapter Seventeen

After nearly freezing while running laps, Dominick and Michael decided that their war against Pusser had run its course. If it continued, they knew something they couldn't come back from would happen to one of them. Pusser wasn't one to grant a truce, but over time, as the pranks grew more distant in the rearview mirror, he relaxed and quit punishing the five of them any more than he did the other Turtles.

In mid-December, Hartfield Academy broke for Christmas. Dominick knew it would be weird returning home. From his family's perspective, he had always been part of them, and it was odd for him to have been kept away for so long. To Dominick, he had only been "home" for a few weeks. Life at the Academy was the new normal for him and his stomach was nervous at the thought of returning.

On December 15th, the stream of cars returned to the academy in mid-morning and continued through the afternoon. Michael Hollister had told Dominick that no one was coming to pick him up, so he'd been put on a bus home early that morning.

Unlike when the entire family came when he arrived at the Academy, it was just Joe in the car when it pulled to a stop.

"Hi, Dad," Dominick said. He waited hesitantly at the curb, unsure of what kind of reaction he was going to get. Things had been very messy at home in the time leading up to his departure to Hartfield.

His father came around the car and grabbed Dominick in a strong embrace. "Nicky, we've missed you, boy." He pulled Dominick back to look at him and rubbed his hand over the close-cropped hair. "I swear you've grown. At least most of you has. No hippies here at Hartfield, eh?"

"No sir."

"That's not a bad thing."

"No, sir."

Joe held him at arm's length for a long moment, then smiled, and said, "C'mon, we've got a long ride home. Your brother had school today, but your Mom and I both took the day off from work. She's home baking mincemeat cookies and making a roast for us. Let's get on the road."

It was several hours past dark when they pulled into the driveway at home. His mother met him on the front porch and gave him a smothering hug, followed by the same inspection Joe had given him. "Oh, Nicky, they cut your beautiful hair! And what are they feeding you? You're skin and bones!"

"They feed me fine, Mom. All I can eat. But they march us and we do calisthenics every day." He patted his non-existent stomach and slipped into a James Cagney accent. "Best shape of my life, Ma."

"Oh, you." She flipped her apron at him. "Come in the house. I've got a surprise for you."

Dominick paused and sniffed the air. "Smells like a mincemeat cookie and pot roast surprise to me."

"Joe, you told him!"

Joe grinned sheepishly and shrugged, then slipped past them into the house.

"Yes, smart boy, I made your favorites."

One step inside the front door, he heard the beating feet of Connie running down the hall. She launched herself at Dominick with a cry of, "Bubby!" Dominick staggered back a step at the impact, but squeezed her tight.

"Hello, Squig. I've missed you."

For the rest of the day, Connie was never far from Dominick.

Sam was the only Davidner not thrilled to see Dominick return. He glanced at him, gave him a slight nod and said, "Hey."

I think he liked having the bedroom to himself. No worry. I'll be back at Hartfield soon enough.

The two weeks of Christmas break passed quickly. On Christmas morning, Dominick opened two new Hardy Boys books, a football, and a canvas army surplus coat. His mother had sewn a name patch on that said, "Davidner." Dominick had to admit the jacket was pretty cool.

That afternoon, they settled into their Christmas dinner, with ham, mashed potatoes, and lasagna. It was one of two meals each year, along with Thanksgiving, where even Sam was allowed to eat until he could eat no more.

Just as he felt settled back into family life again, it was time to return to the Academy.

Again, it was just Joe and Dominick on the trip. Dominick had been nervous on the trip down, afraid that he would feel like an outsider, but he had worried unnecessarily.

No matter what, no matter how stupid we are, or how much we screw up, family is still family, and home is where they have to take you in.

A hundred miles of pavement rolled under their wheels in silence. Finally, Dominick said, "Dad?"

"Mmm-hmm," Joe answered without taking his eyes off the road.

"How much did it cost to fix Mr. Bratski's shed and stuff?"

Joe glanced at him with a slight smile, a few months' time had given a little distance and perspective. "Oh, there was no fixing that shed. You sent it to the great shed graveyard in the sky."

"You know what I mean. I just want to know how bad I messed up."

"Well, we had to buy him a new shed, which was almost a hundred and fifty dollars. Mr. Bratski is a nice man, though. He's been letting us make payments to him."

Dominick's cheeks reddened. *Oh, that's great. Mom and Dad's budget is already stretched to the limit, and I'm just adding to it.*

"There was no saving his rose garden, though. You tore through those pretty damn good. Next summer, when you're home, I've volunteered you to help Mr. Bratski with his lawn and hedges and also to try and rebuild his rose garden."

Dominick absorbed that and nodded. "Good. That will be good. Dad, I'm sorry about the money. I'll pay you back as soon as I can. There's just no way for me to earn money while I'm at the Academy."

Joe didn't say anything in reply, but didn't turn the offer down.

"I just kind of ... I don't know, I guess I lost my way for a while there. I'm back on track now."

"I swear, Nicky, sometimes you sound like yourself, and sometimes you sound like an adult. Which reminds me. I don't suppose you noticed while you were home, but I've quit chewing tobacco. It saves us a little money, and you just might be right about it being dangerous."

Dominick hadn't noticed, but he felt a load lighten inside him. His father had developed black spots on his inner lip in 1975. Numerous surgeries had followed, taking out parts of his lip and tongue, but none of it had stopped the spread of the cancer. It had killed him in 1979.

Maybe it's not too late, Dad.

Dominick looked out the window and was quiet until he fell asleep. He didn't wake up until Joe stopped the car in the circular drive at Hartfield Academy.

Chapter Eighteen

The turbulent, cultural earthquake that was 1967 and '68 in America passed Dominick Davidner by without leaving a mark. When he had first arrived in his family's home in August 1966, he hadn't been able to find his center. He had no idea how to be a forty-year-old man, stuck in a child's body. That imbalance had led him to be banished to Hartfield Academy.

There were other people who seemed as strange as he felt at Hartfield. Especially Michael Hollister, who Dominick had come to believe might be in the same predicament he was in. Over the first two years he spent at Hartfield, pieces of the puzzle had fit together. Michael's preternatural perspective on events as they happened and his genius achievements in the classroom—but more than anything, there was a natural bond Dominick felt with Michael—a brotherhood he had never felt with Sam.

In the summers, away from Hartfield, Dominick committed to being an ideal son to his parents. He told them he didn't want an allowance any more—he wanted to earn his own money. The first summer back, he took over lawn mowing responsibilities from Sam, which pleased his older brother no end.

He also mowed Mr. Bratski's lawn and trimmed his hedges, still trying to make up for his misadventure from the summer before. A few weeks into mowing the Bratski's lawn, their mower choked to a halt and wouldn't start again.

"Huh. Looks like you're off the hook for today, Nicky," Mr. Bratski said. Despite their near-collision and the damage to his beloved roses, Ivan Bratski liked Dominick. "I'll have to load it in the trunk and take it down to Wilson's Small Engine shop."

"Oh, don't do that, Mr. Bratski. Do you mind if I take it home so my Dad and I can look it over?"

"Oh, sure, fine. I guess I won't be able to take it in until tomorrow, anyway."

That night, Dominick and Joe tore the engine apart, tuned it up and made it purr. Dominick did his best to pretend not to know what he was doing, but Joe had to admit he had clever hands, and his small fingers were able to fit into spaces that Joe couldn't.

The next day, Dominick proudly rolled the mower across the street. Mr. Bratski came out with a slight grin, cradling his china coffee cup, and said, "Give up?"

Dominick answered by yanking the pull chord in one smooth motion. The engine fired and idled smoothly. Mr. Bratski's eyebrows shot up. "She didn't sound that good the day I brought 'er home from Sears! You've got a talent, young man."

"My Dad did it. I just helped."

The next week, when Dominick returned to mow the Bratski's lawn again, there was another mower sitting next to the shed.

"That's Dimitri's mower, from down the block. He says he can't get it running. Want to give it a try?"

Just like that, Davidner and Son's Small Engine Repair became a viable business. Five or six times a week, someone would show up in their driveway with an old mower in the trunk. Initially, some people were reluctant to leave their mower or rototiller off with a kid, but as their reputation spread, that concern evaporated.

The business helped Dominick begin building a little nest egg for his future plans, all of which revolved around Emily, and gave him the chance to pay back part of the money he had cost his parents.

More than any of that, though, was the opportunity to spend long hours in the shop with his father, listening to him whistle under his breath, mumbling, and at the end of another project, saying, "Give 'er a go, Nicky."

The next summer, there were mowers lined up outside the shop when he returned from Hartfield Academy, and they never stopped appearing. Dominick gave up on the appearance that his Dad did all the work and just set to work every morning. It made the business of being a middle-aged man in a child's body more tolerable, and the time passed more quickly.

Plus, the scholarship he had been offered at Hartfield was only good for the first two years. If he wanted to go again, he needed to earn enough money to be able to help his parents cover the extra outlay.

All summer, as he worked, he planned.

Get through Hartfield Academy and graduate. Then I'll be eighteen. I should have enough money saved up from fixing engines that I can buy a car and begin my search for Emily.

Dominick had managed not to mention Emily to anyone, but she was never far from his mind.

During that second summer, Dominick often thought of Michael Hollister, as well. The more he thought, the more he came to the conclusion that Michael might be exactly what Dominick himself was—a soul relocated in time, for some unknown purpose. He came to the decision that when he saw him again, at the start of their third year at Hartfield, he would find a way to broach the subject.

The summer of 1970 flew by in a never-ending parade of long days bent over lawnmowers, and before he knew it, Dominick and Joe were back in the car for another trip to Hartfield.

When they passed the Shell station just before the academy, Joe turned to Dominick, and ruffled his hair, which had grown out quickly over the summer. "Ready to go under the razor for another year?"

"Yeah. I don't mind it. Easy to take care of it, that way, and it saves on my comb budget."

"I'll really miss you, Nicky. I know why we started this whole business with the Academy, and it was important at the time, but now, I don't know ... "

"I know, Dad, and I'm glad. Back then, I thought maybe I didn't deserve to be in the family anymore. I know that's not true, now. But I started something at Hartfield. I have brothers here, now, too, and they depend on me. I can't just leave and let them down."

"I only want you to know it's up to you."

"Thanks, Dad. Gotta finish what I started, though, right?"

Joe turned down the long driveway and onto the broad, circular driveway. As soon as they pulled to a stop, Dominick saw Michael Hollister standing on the curb, waiting for him. He looked at his father.

Joe smiled. "Okay, I get it. When you're twelve years old, nothing is more important than your friends. Go on. I'll be here to pick you up for Christmas."

"Love you, Dad," Dominick said, and clambered over the backseat to get his knapsack, then jumped out the back door.

"What's up, genius?" he shouted at Michael, who was only a few feet away.

Michael smiled. "Nothin', hothead. It's been a long, boring summer around here without you to help me get into trouble."

Dominick and Michael had never really talked about what Michael's home situation was, but since that first Christmas, Dominick knew Michael had never gone back. It had surprised Dominick when he learned that Michael was from Middle Falls, Oregon, since that was where Dominick himself had been living when he had been shot and killed. Eventually, he had put it down to a cosmic coincidence.

Dominick smiled and slapped Michael on the shoulder. "We'll have to see what we can do about that!"

Dominick looked at a frightened first year, clinging to his mother and shook his head. "No way we were that scrawny when we got here." He stopped, gave an appraising look up and down at Michael, who was at the beginning of a growth spurt. "Well, maybe you, Hollister."

Michael straightened up to attention and said, "Don't look now, Dom, but I might have you by half an inch or so."

"You might end up taller, but let's face it. You're always gonna be slow."

"Slow? You know that's no insult to a Turtle!" Michael snapped his fingers, "Oh, hey, you know what we get to do this year, right?"

Dominick rubbed his chin. "Torture another prefect?"

"Well, yeah, obviously. But mostly, we finally get to play in the Game."

Dominick nodded. He had forgotten all about the Hartfield Game, where all the classes competed against each other. "It'll be our first year, though. You know we're gonna be meat."

Michael shrugged, then flashed his sly smile. "Maybe, maybe not. I had a lot of time to think and poke around the Academy this summer. I think I've got a plan."

Dominick looked around and acted like he was speaking to an audience. "And this, ladies and gentlemen, is why I like having a genius for a best friend."

Michael just shook his head.

They walked away from the front lawn, toward the barracks. When they were out of earshot of all the other cadets, Dominick said, "There's something I've wanted to talk to you about all summer."

"Yeah?"

"Yeah." *Crap. Why do I start things and then wish I hadn't?* "I know this is going to sound weird, but, do you believe in ghosts?"

An odd expression crossed Michael's face—part dread, part fascination. "I didn't used to, but I guess I do now. That's a weird thing to think about all summer. Did you see a ghost in your house?"

"No, not really. It's just ... I know you're going to think I'm crazy—"

"—I already do—"

Dominick punched him gently in the shoulder. "—but I kind of feel ... like I'm a ghost."

Michael stopped. Even though no one was nearby, he lowered his voice and said, "What are you talking about?"

Now that I'm here, I have no idea how to explain it. What can I say? "It's hard to explain. It's like I've lived this life before."

"Like reincarnation, or something?"

Does living the same life over again count as reincarnation, or would that mean I show up as someone else... Or maybe a cat? I wish I knew. Dominick opened his mouth to say something, but stopped. *What the hell. There's just no way to explain this, is there?* He opened his mouth again, but shut it, frustrated. "You know what? Never mind. It's too damn weird. So, tell me about how we're going to win the Hartfield Game as first-year players."

Michael wasn't one to be easily put off a scent. He still hadn't moved, and stared at Dominick long and hard. *I can tell he wants to ask me more, but he won't. He never snoops into my life, and expects the same in return. I'm good with that.*

Finally, Michael looked away and shrugged, a gesture that said, *Okay, if that's the way you want it.*

"I've been working on strategy all summer. Here's what I think we need to do..."

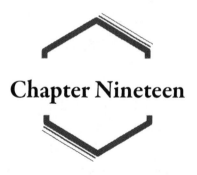

Chapter Nineteen

The Hartfield Game was held the third week of October, and all cadets who were Third Year or older participated. The rules were deceptively simple. Every cadet was given a flag belt, and they were in the game until an opposing player pulled their flag, or until an opposing player pulled their Flag Bearer's flag. The teams played on until only one team had a Flag Bearer still in the game, and that team was the victor.

The Third Year cadets were only eleven or twelve years old, though, while the Tenth Years were seventeen or eighteen, nearly full-grown, and ready to go into further military academies or the armed forces. It was typically a slaughter for the third and fourth year classes. No Third Year class had ever finished higher than 4th, but no other class had the advantage of having Michael Hollister.

The first week of October, Michael took Dominick for a walk at the back of academy, along the ocean cliff that marked the western border of the school. To the south was a dense wood that was dark and foreboding. They walked along the cliff's edge, and Michael gestured out over the Pacific, then pointed down at a trail that crisscrossed down about forty feet, then dead-ended.

"Stand here with me for a minute and look down at the trail, like we're making a plan. I don't think any of the upperclassmen are worried about us, but in case they're watching, I don't want to give them an idea."

Dominick nodded and followed the direction Michael was pointing with his eyes. They stood there for several minutes, then casually walked to the point where the woods and the cliff intersected. Michael led Dominick thirty feet back from the cliff, then stepped onto a small game trail and disappeared. Inside the dense woods, it was dark and quiet, as the near-ceaseless winds that came off the Pacific couldn't penetrate the trees and underbrush.

"Come on," Michael said, breaking into a jog. They moved a hundred yards along the trail, then Michael stopped. "Here. Look around. What do you see?"

Dominick looked down at the trail, up at the trees, and along the ledge of a rock wall that marked the southern border of the campus.. "I don't see much of anything."

Michael smiled, a rare expression on his face, which softened his sometimes stern demeanor. "Exactly."

There were long hanging vines that dropped down the face of the rock wall, and Michael stuck his arm right through the vines, then gently swept them back.

"It's a cave!"

"Yes. Not much of a cave, and it doesn't lead anywhere, but I don't think anyone on campus knows about it. The Third Years always get picked off early because we're smaller and slower. That's why they always look for a place to hide, but the upperclassmen know all the hiding spots. I've been looking through all the records of the history of the Hartfield Game in the library, and there's never been mention of a cave. I don't think anyone's ever stumbled on this place."

"Except you, Genius."

Michael shrugged. "When I first got here, I spent a lot of time walking around the grounds, trying to get the lay of the land. I came upon this place by accident, and I've just been saving it. We'll only be able to use it once, though, so should we use it this year, or save it?"

Dominick took a moment and let the possibilities run through his head. "This will give us our only chance of survival, and it would be so cool if we won as First Years. I think we should go for it."

"Okay. Since the Turtles elected me Captain—"

"—of course—"

"—I've got to write our strategy up in advance and turn it in to Captain Peterson."

"Okay, who's our flag bearer?"

"You're the fastest Turtle, Dom, so it would make sense to be you. But, I need a second in command in case I get captured early. I want that to be you. No one else is very fast, but I think we can count on Will to keep his head."

Dominick held back several of the vines and poked his head into the small cave. A strong smell of an old animal kill filled his nostrils. "Ugh, not gonna be too much fun hanging out in there for a few hours, is it?"

"Better than being picked off and finishing last. We can bring a bucket out here, so we can relieve ourselves."

"How about flashlights?"

"We can have them, but we won't use them in the cave. They'll give us away."

"You've thought of everything."

"Few battle plans survive first contact with the enemy, but I'm trying to think of all contingencies."

Dominick squinted at Michael in the growing darkness. *What kid talks like that? What's going on with you, Michael? Who are you, really?*

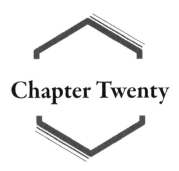

Chapter Twenty

The day of the Hartfield Game was cool and blustery, but not as bitterly cold as late October on the northern California coast could sometimes be. Heavy gray clouds hung low in the sky, threatening to add precipitation during the game at some point.

Inside the Turtles' barrack, Michael pulled his team into a tight semi-circle at the very back, near the restrooms. Their prefect for the year was an earnest Tenth Year named Doug Brant. The prefects that had come after Pusser were a bit of a let-down, in terms of entertainment value, and Doug was the quietest yet.

Michael leaned in close to the gathered Turtles and said, in a voice barely above a whisper, "It's not that I don't trust Brant. It's that I don't trust anyone who's not a Turtle."

Strong nods from every Turtle.

Smart, Hollister. Establish Us vs. Them. Great way to build a team.

"Here's how it's going to work. The older teams will call a truce with each other, just long enough to get rid of us, the fourth and the fifth years. That way they don't have to worry about us. They're bigger than us, faster than us, and they have experience that we don't. Essentially, they're better than us in every way."

"So, no problem then, right? We've got this," Dominick said, which broke the tension, and the Turtles laughed.

"We've got one advantage, and that's sheer numbers. There are nineteen of us – more than any other class. But the only way to maintain that advantage is to keep our numbers intact. And to do that we need to hide. The problem is, they know all the hiding spots. All except one. When Commander Hartfield starts the game, follow me to the cliff."

Uncertain nods came from all sides. Even the Turtles knew that once you hid on the cliff, there was nowhere to run, but they trusted Michael.

Quietly, Michael said, "Who are we?"

The group answered, equally as quiet, "The Turtles."

Michael stood, raised his voice, "Who are we?"

The group around him stood as one, shouting, "We are the Turtles, the mighty, mighty Turtles!"

WHEN THE TURTLES REACHED the cliff, they veered off to the left, single file, along the path that Michael had showed Dominick a few weeks before. They quickly arrived at the sheer rock wall with the heavy vines hanging down.

Michael and Dominick turned around, faced the rest of the Turtles.

"Well, here we are," Dominick said, with a grin.

"Hollister, I don't mean to complain, but this is our great plan? To stand in the middle of a trail and wait for them to come take us down?" Will Summers asked.

Other Turtles were not so kind.

"We're dead."

"Can you hear anyone coming?"

"Crap, I thought you had a plan, Michael."

With a theatrical flair, Michael pushed his hand through the vines and pulled them aside enough that the boys could see what was behind them. "Voila," Michael said.

"Whoa," Billy Guenther said, almost in a whisper.

"Yeah, whoa," Dominick said. "I told you Michael had a plan."

"Are we just going to hide in there?" Billy asked. It was obvious that he, and a number of other Turtles, didn't relish a day spent in the dank cave.

Michael and Dominick nodded.

"Are there flashlights in there, at least?"

"No, dummy," Dominick answered. "When they figure out we've disappeared, they're gonna come looking for us in the forest. They'll see a light through the vines."

"So, we're just gonna hide in there all day?"

"That's the plan," Michael said. "Eventually, they'll get tired of looking for us, and whatever alliances they've formed will fall apart. If we get lucky, they'll weaken each other enough, so we can swoop in and overwhelm whoever's left with our numbers."

Billy and several other Turtles looked uncertain.

"It's either that," Michael said, "or we go out and face the Hawks, Eagles, and Badgers head-on."

"Yeah, then we'll finish last, just like every other first-year team," Dominick said. "Is that what you want?"

No answer.

"Come on, then, Turtles." Michael was the first into the cave, followed by Dominick and the rest of the unit. The cave was cramped, and smelled of long-rotting animal kills.

Terry Jordan scrunched his nose and looked around. "Ugh, so awful! What is that smell?"

"That's the decaying bodies of the last unit to hide in here. They never made it out alive," Dominick said. "You're next."

"Listen, I know it's not perfect," Michael said. "Dom and I did what we could to get it ready in here. There are buckets that you can sit on if you get tired of standing, but I don't recommend sitting on the floor of the cave. It's pretty gross. And there's a bucket in the corner if you have to relieve yourself. Other than that, stand still, be quiet, and wait."

"How long?"

"At least until dark. By then, they'll be pretty frantic. They'll think we caught a bus into Crescent City or something."

Like their namesake, the Turtles pulled their heads into the shell of the cave and waited. They stood or sat noiselessly for more than an hour before they heard the first group of predators looking for them. That first group passed by at a walking pace, chattering and cutting up, talking about home, and the girls in town.

The waiting went on. Michael and Dominick had known it would be tough to huddle together as noiselessly as possible in the small cave, but anticipating it and actually living it were different things. The hardest part for all of them was the cold. It had started raining in the middle of the afternoon. That helped the marine air wick through their coats and settle into their bones. And, sitting or standing for long periods, moving as little as possible, left them stiff and sore.

Yet still, they waited.

Michael and Dominick held whispered conversations, when they were sure no other teams were on the trail.

"They've got to be getting frantic about now," Dominick said.

Michael smiled in the darkness. "Their alliance is one of convenience, so I don't expect it to hold for too long. I bet they're already hunting each other, just to have something to do, and to gain an advantage for the end game."

A little after 5:00, more than five hours after the Game had started, a serious group of boys came hunting them. Four upperclassmen, walking slowly, looking under every rock and behind every tree. They followed the game trail that passed in front of the cave and passed by so close that one of their shoulders brushed against the hanging vines, causing them to swing and sway a bit.

Inside, the Turtles held their breath. This was the moment of truth.

The boys passed on by, but the boy who had brushed the vines stopped and cocked his head. He took two steps back toward the cave opening. He poked at the vines and his hand passed through them, into nothing but darkness.

His fingers came within an inch of touching Michael's shoulder, but everyone in the cave silently leaned back a few inches, just out of range.

The boy said, "Huh!" and stood thoughtfully on the trail, looking at his hand, as though it might have passed into another dimension and returned. The rest of his group continued walking forward. "Hang on, guys," the boy called out, "I think there might be something here." He reached out and tentatively touched the vines, which swayed at his touch. With a flourish, he grabbed the left-most vine and swept his hand to the right, revealing the cave, and the nineteen Turtles hiding there.

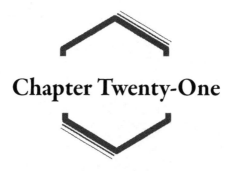

Chapter Twenty-One

"Holy shit!" the boy cried. "We found 'em!"

From the depths of the cave, the nineteen Turtles poured out like ants on a forgotten picnic, swarming the bigger boys under their combined weight. With a war whoop, they took them to the ground.

The leader of the hunters tried to yell, "We found 'em!" at the top of his lungs, but with the weight of half a dozen Turtles on his chest, the words did not carry. In seconds, the younger boys had pulled the flags of the four older ones, ending their game.

Michael, breathing hard with excitement, said, "According to the rules of the Game, you are dead and are not allowed to communicate with your unit."

Dominick saw that one of the older boys held a Turtle flag firmly in his grasp and looked around to see who they had lost.

Billy Guenther stepped forward and raised his hand.

"Billy," Michael said, "it's not that I don't trust the honor of these fine Badgers, but make sure they don't communicate with anyone else on the way to the library. We're going to rebuild the vines as best we can and stay right here until full dark."

The five vanquished boys, four large and one small, headed down the trail for the school. Yet only four of them walked dejectedly with their heads down.

When they had disappeared down the trail. Michael said, "Okay, we're not really staying here, but here's what we're gonna do. Freddy, you stay here in the cave, hidden as best you can. We're going to be on the move. If someone is about to capture you here, scream at the top of your lungs how many of them there are. Got it?"

Freddy nodded.

Dominick and the rest of the boys did the best they could to repair the damage that had been done to the vines, to make it look like Turtles might still be hiding inside.

With that done, the Turtles jogged down the path for fifty yards, until they came to a spot where the underbrush closed in and the trail was pinched down by large rocks on either side, causing them to walk in single file.

The Turtles divided themselves, with half of them hiding behind the rock on either side of the trail, leaving Michael as bait in the middle. They didn't have to wait long before they heard Freddy scream "Four," before he fell silent.

Michael kneeled down on the trail, as though he was tying his shoe, unaware of the impending danger. Almost immediately, four Badgers came at a full run. The leader saw Michael, apparently vulnerable on the trail in front of them and screamed, "There he is!"

Michael feigned surprise, said, "Oh, crap," and turned to run away, but stumbled and fell. He crawled away from the boys on his hands and knees.

"Wait a minute," the lead boy said, squinting into the falling darkness. "Is this the little shit that's supposed to be so smart? He don't look like much to—"

Before he could finish his sentence, the Turtles swarmed again. The Badgers were so surprised, they went down without taking a single Turtle with them.

Dominick turned to Michael and said, "We'll trade four for one all day, but how long do we think they'll keep falling for it?"

"I don't think this routine will work anymore. The Badgers we just trapped will find a way to get word to everyone. We'll have to find a different plan."

The Turtles set off down the path, then veered off onto another, more obscure animal trail that Michael and Dominick had scouted out. A few yards off the main trail, they found where a huge tree had fallen and had lodged itself against a boulder and in the lower branches of two neighboring trees.

"This spot was too obvious during the day," Michael whispered, "but I think we'll be okay here for a few minutes, now that it's mostly dark." He laid a hand on Dominick's shoulder. "Dom, you're our fastest. Make a scouting run, but don't be gone too long. If you're not back in thirty minutes, we'll assume you're dead and make a new plan."

Dominick smiled and headed back to the main trail. He wound his way down it, toward the cliff, trying to strike the best balance he could between speed and silence.

Damn, this is fun. Who knew playing a kid's game could be this exhilarating?

He came to the edge of the forest that bordered the cliff and dropped down onto a ledge where he could stick his head up over the edge. He saw two boys in the far corner, huddled down in a depression. Michael had been right. Their flashlights only served to give them away.

Dominick slipped up over the edge of the cliff in the covering darkness and made his way back to the forest.

Only two people in evidence. I expected more.

He jogged more quickly now, less worried about stumbling into a marauding patrol of upper classmen. He found the edge of the forest where it ran parallel to the great lawn at the front of the school. He hid behind an oak tree and peered out. Again, two boys, this time standing at the flag pole, silhouetted from behind by the lights that pointed up at the flags.

Andy Tanner and Bob Morgan. Figures. Andy's the fastest runner in the school, so of course he's their flag bearer. I'll never be able to run him down.

Dominick slipped back into the cover of the forest, then moved silently to the nearest building – the staff quarters. There were no lights on inside the building and it gave him perfect cover as he slid along the back of it.

Where are all the other classes?

Dominick moved noiselessly between the buildings, but couldn't find a sign of anyone.

Gonna have to take a chance. I might get captured, but I don't know enough to report back yet.

There was a tall row of hedges that surrounded the main building of the academy, which held the great hall, Commander Hartfield's office, and the library, where all the vanquished players would be.

The rules of the game said that an active player couldn't go inside any of the buildings, but there was no rule about hiding behind the hedges. Dominick edged behind them and moved toward the long windows of the library. He reached the nearest one and slowly peeked around the corner.

The room was brightly lit, with a table holding cookies, hot cider, and hot chocolate. Much more importantly, the library was full of cadets. Dominick dropped his head away and closed his eyes, trying to take a mental picture of how many cadets he had seen.

The answer he came up with astounded him. *All of them. It looks like all of them are already in there. Holy shit, that means that those four I saw out there, and all the Turtles hiding in the woods, are the last players remaining. We could actually win this!*

Dominick glanced at his watch. *My half hour's almost up. They'll think I've been captured.* Abandoning all attempts at quiet, Dominick jumped out of the hedge and ran straight for the trail he had followed. *Even if they see me, I've got a big enough head start, I can lead them right back to a trap where we can overpower them with sheer numbers.*

He tore across the grass and into the welcoming embrace of the deep forest. He paused and looked back over his shoulder. No one was following him.

Good. Probably would have killed myself again trying to follow this rabbit trail in the dark.

He set off at a steady jog. After a few minutes, he arrived at the two rocks that pinched the trail.

Damn. Passed that little turn off in the dark. Gonna have to be more careful.

He backtracked fifty paces, and found the spur trail. He turned onto it, and in a few more steps, he was at the fallen tree.

"Good news?" Michael asked.

Dominick's face split in a grin that could be seen even in the dark. He held up his hand, and bent over double to catch his breath. "They must have gotten tired of depleting themselves by sending scout teams after us, so they went after each other. There's only two teams left, and two people on each of them. I snuck over and looked in the library window. You won't believe it—everyone's in there just waiting for the game to finish."

Michael pumped his hand once. "That's exactly what I was hoping for. Do you know where the last two teams are?"

"Well, I know where they *were*. The two Badgers are just hanging around the flagpole. I think they're counting on the fact that Andy can outrun anyone in the school."

Michael nodded, thoughtfully. He looked at Dominick. "Any chance you could catch him?"

"None at all." *If I had another few years to grow, maybe. But right now? No way, brother.*

"Who's the other team?"

"The Hawks. They're both hanging out back at the track."

"Good. We'll have to expose Will to attract them, but it's worth the risk."

"Let's go."

When they arrived back at the edge of the forest, Michael said, "Will, here's all you do. Try to creep along the edge of the forest, like you're scared. Maybe limp a little. Hopefully, they'll see you and come after you."

"It's dark," Will said. "I don't think they'll see me."

Michael fished in his pocket. "That's what I've been saving this for." He handed Will a flashlight. "Don't be too obvious with it, right? Just flash it on the ground ahead of you, like you're looking for a trail or something. They'll see you and come after you. We'll be right behind you, and we'll strip them of their flags as they run by us."

Will eased out into the grass, wet with the remainder of the afternoon's rain. They hadn't needed to worry about the Hawks spotting Will. They were on the lookout and saw him almost immediately.

One of the Hawks illuminated Will with his flashlight. Then another flashlight beam, and another, and another.

Hiding just at the edge of the forest, Michael whispered, "I thought there were only two Hawks left?"

"I guess I missed them," Dominick answered.

"Will," Michael hissed. "Run toward us, now!"

He didn't need to say it twice. Will sprinted toward the rest of the Turtles, the safety of the forest. He was not the fastest runner, though, and the older Hawks closed the gap between them quickly.

Everything was moving too fast. They would never be able to stop the older boys at the speed they were running, especially since there were four of them instead of only two. They would just blow right through the Turtles, run Will down, and strip him of his flag. So close, and yet so far.

Will ran right past them, just like he was supposed to. The Hawks were only a few yards behind, just enough distance that Michael had time to throw his body across the trail. The first Hawk never saw him, stepped onto the small of his back, twisted his ankle, and went flying off into the bushes. The second sensed a commotion and tried to slow, but it was too late. He tripped over Michael and went sprawling onto the path. The third and fourth boys did the same.

"Dom, get 'em!" Michael hollered.

The Turtles jumped on the boys and stripped them of their flags.

When they sorted out all the arms, legs, and torsos, all four Hawks were without their flag. Michael untangled himself, stood up, and started to give an order, when one of the Hawks held his flag aloft. For the purposes of the game, Michael was dead.

Dominick and Michael exchanged a glance. Michael had gotten them this far, now it was up to Dominick to take down the strongest and the fastest.

Michael and the vanquished Hawks walked out of the woods and across the track toward the library. Dominick hunkered down with the remaining Turtles.

"We've got them outnumbered pretty badly, but we still want to be cautious. If we rush them, Andy will just outrun all of us, and I'm not sure we'll ever catch him. That will make for a long night. Everyone surround Will, so if they jump us, they'll have a hard time getting to him. Follow me."

Dominick turned his flashlight on, using the single beam to illuminate the path that wound through the woods toward the front of the school. When he saw the lights around the flagpole, he switched it off.

The two older boys were still standing in the middle of the great lawn, where it was impossible to sneak up on them. Dominick tapped his fingers against the flashlight, thinking.

How the heck do we use our numbers to beat their strength and speed? Maybe I'm just making it too complicated.

Mind made up, he turned to the fourteen remaining Turtles and said, "Here's what we're gonna do. Pretend there's a big clock face covering the lawn ..."

Five minutes later, the Turtles were in place, hiding in as many locations surrounding the lawn as was possible given the cover, with Will Summers left behind in the forest. Dominick whistled once - sharp and short. The Turtles emerged from their hiding spots and walked slowly toward the two older boys at the flagpoles.

This is it. This is their chance. If they run right now, they'll break through us easily, and we'll be hunting them all night.

The Turtles approached slowly, but methodically. Dominick had guessed that if they came out of hiding and rushed at the Tenth Years, it would have spooked them. Instead, they moved simultaneously at a half-march, which ended up confusing the older boys.

The boys from the opposing team didn't run, but instead stayed in place, turning this way, then that, watching the jaws of the trap slowly close around them. Bob Morgan was caught in a web of indecision, unable to decide whether to attack, or flee. In the end, that indecision made either impossible.

The noose of Turtles closed around them until there were no gaps to escape through. Finally, Andy Tanner said, "I'm gonna make a run for it," and ran straight toward the woods. That was where Dominick had placed himself. He wasn't fast enough to keep up with Andy, but he was good at judging distance, speed, and velocity.

Andy juked left, then right, but Dominick stayed focused on his mid-section. Just when it appeared Andy might slip away, Dominick launched himself at Andy's feet. Andy jumped, trying to hurdle him to freedom, but Dominick's shoulder caught his boots and the older boy tumbled to the ground. The Turtles on either side of Dominick jumped into action, and jumped on Andy, pinning him before he could escape.

Dominick recovered his balance, rolled over and pulled the flag from Andy's belt.

The 50th annual Hartfield Game was over, and the Turtles were the victors.

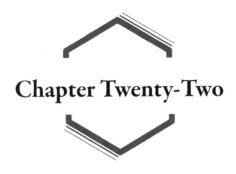

Chapter Twenty-Two

Dominick and the rest of the Turtles followed the defeated Badgers into the library. The door swung open and the room hushed. When everyone inside saw the expression on Bob and Andy's face, a buzz started at the front and spread.

Michael Hollister stood and looked at Dominick, who smiled widely and threw his arms up in a sign of total victory. Michael and the other captured Turtles erupted in a cheer, and soon there was a circle of jumping, yelling Turtles celebrating while the other classes looked on.

"Settle down now, cadets, settle down," Commander Hartfield's voice rang out. The Turtles quieted down, but stood together, arms slung around each other's shoulders, grinning like drunken fools.

"Come in, Turtles, come in. Have a seat here at the front table. It is reserved for the victors."

The Badgers had already been gathering there, expecting the inevitable victory, even when outnumbered so badly, and now they moved away, clearing space. The Turtles sat down, Michael in the middle, with Dominick and Will on either side.

Commander Hartfield cleared his throat, and all cadets turned toward him. "It's been a momentous day, hasn't it? Congratulations to all the cadets, from the first captured to the final ones standing. You fought with honor, and that is the most important thing of all."

Captain Peterson, standing at the back of the room, applauded, and with seeming reluctance, the rest of the cadets joined in.

THE DEATH AND LIFE OF DOMINICK DAVIDNER   113

"And in the end, there were only Turtles standing. In the fifty-year history of the Hartfield Game, no team competing in their first year has ever won. Hell, let's be honest: none has ever come close. All rise, please, and salute the victors!"

The rest of the cadets shuffled to their feet, faced the Turtles and snapped off a salute.

"As is our tradition, I've had Lieutenant Ignovich make a feast worthy of the day. Please proceed to the mess hall."

The feast turned out to be worthy indeed. Roasted turkey with dressing, and both pumpkin and apple pies for dessert made for a Thanksgiving celebration a month early.

It wouldn't have mattered if they had served Meals Ready to Eat from the supply closet, as far as the Turtles were concerned. It still would have been a meal of celebration. They had done what had been thought to be impossible.

As Michael tucked in to his dinner, Dominick leaned over and said, "The Turtles are great, but we never would have come close without you, Genius."

Michael's cheeks turned a little red, but he just turned to Dominick and said, "This is cool, but we're going to have to get everybody back to the barracks soon. Reveille still sounds at oh six hundred, no matter how late we stay up."

I swear, you're an old man in a child's body. When are you ever going to learn to relax and revel in the moment?

After the meal, the Turtles headed back to their barrack at Michael's encouragement and within minutes were stripped down and on their bunks. The exertion of the day, combined with the emotional victory and the tryptophan in the turkey, quickly knocked them out.

Dominick and Michael lay on their bunks, quietly dissecting the strategy of the day and talking about a plan for the following year's Hartfield Game. They were just discussing whether it would be possible for them to win every Game they played in, when Billy Guenther, whose bunk was at the front of the room, shouted, "Officer present!"

All Turtles, even those who had been dead asleep a moment before, scrambled to their feet and did their best to stand at attention. Captain Peterson said, "At ease," then walked straight to the back, where Dominick and Michael were.

"Cadets Hollister and Davidner. Get dressed immediately."

Dominick and Michael scrambled for their clothes and threw them on. As soon as they slipped their boots on, Peterson said, "Follow me."

Dominick looked a question at Michael, who only shrugged in return.

Gotta be something pretty bad to yank us out of bed at lights out, especially after the day we just had. If something had happened back home, though, why would they have needed Michael too? I guess all will be revealed shortly.

Peterson led the boys into the main hall and ushered them into Commander Hartfield's office.

Inside, there were three Badgers: Doug Brant, their prefect, along with Bob Morgan and Andy Tanner. The three of them were held at attention.

Hartfield indicated two chairs opposite his desk and said, "Sit down, cadets"

Michael and Dominick sat, appearing very small in the chairs in front of the massive desk.

"I have a few questions I'm going to ask you, but before I do, there are a few things we need to talk about. What you boys accomplished today was remarkable—something to be proud of. However, if you look at our flag," he nodded his head toward the Hartfield flag displayed behind him, "you'll see there are three words on it: Honor. Brotherhood. Duty. 'Honor' is the first word, because without our honor, there can be no true victory. If we lose our honor, we lose ourselves. Understood?"

Michael and Dominick nodded.

This feels bad. I think it's a setup.

"Good. Now. These three officers of the Badgers have come forth with a serious accusation, and it is important that you tell me the truth. If you do, there will be repercussions, but the situation will be salvageable." Hartfield glanced down at a folder in front of him, then said, "The Badgers are maintaining that the Turtles won by cheating today."

Michael nearly jumped out of his chair. "Bullshit!"

Hartfield fixed him with a gaze as calm as could be. His voice remained steady. "This will be your only warning, Cadet Hollister. You will sit and listen, and you will not speak unless I ask you a question."

Michael sat back down, but Dominick could feel the steam coming off him.

At the side of the room, Bob Morgan smirked.

There's our perpetrator, then. The man with the plan.

"Now, the Badgers are claiming that the Turtles stole their strategic planning guide and used it to win the war. What do you say to that, Cadet Hollister?"

Keep it together, Michael. Losing your cool now won't do us any good.

"Sir, we did not cheat in any way. We never saw their guide." Michael looked directly at Bob Morgan. "Think about it, sir. Their strategy was to put the fastest cadet in the school in the middle of the biggest cadets in the Game and then stand by the flagpole. I didn't need to steal anything to unwind that particular mystery."

Morgan's cheeks turned red, and Dominick thought he heard Captain Peterson stifle a laugh behind them.

"True enough. However, if you had taken their guide prior to the Game today, you would have known just how ham-handed and strategically inept their plan would be."

Hartfield turned his attention to Dominick. "What do you have to say, Cadet Davidner?"

"We didn't cheat, sir. We didn't need to. Michael had been planning this for years. We didn't rely on being bigger or faster, we just relied on being smarter than them, which we were."

"Based on the outcome, I tend not to disagree with that, cadet." Hartfield turned sideways in his chair and stared at the three Badgers standing against the window. "What proof do you bring? I'm not going to convict these cadets of cheating on your word alone."

Morgan coughed slightly, then said, "Lieutenant. Brant, the Turtles' prefect, brought this to my attention, sir."

Hartfield focused on Brant. "Cadet?"

Brant looked like he'd rather be in line for a proctology exam, but said, "Yes, sir. After lights-out two nights ago, I was doing my final check, and when I passed Cadet Davidner's bunk, I noticed a piece of paper sticking out from under his mattress. Initially, I was concerned it might be some type of contraband, so I looked closer and saw that it was just a few sheets of paper. Technically, I knew the cadets should not stash anything under their mattress, but it was a minor point, so I let it go."

"And ..." Hartfield said.

"And, that was it. Until tonight. After the Game was over, I skipped dinner and was first back into the barrack. Something about what I had seen the night before stuck in my head. I went to Cadet Davidner's bunk, lifted it up, and found this, sir." Brant reached in his back pocket and pulled a sheaf of folded pages. He took two steps and handed them to Hartfield.

Hartfield accepted the pages, unfolded them and smoothed them out on the desk in front of him. He glanced up at Michael and

Dominick. "This is, indeed, the strategic plan for the Badgers." He looked at Morgan again and added, "Such as they are. Cadet Davidner, what do you have to say?"

"Sir? I don't know, sir. I have never seen that before in my life. If it was under my mattress, I have no idea how it got there."

"Cadet Hollister?"

"Sir, I have never seen that, either. I think it's a setup. I think they didn't like being beaten by a first-year team, and this is their way of getting back at us."

"Those are serious accusations, cadet, as is the one facing you. Captain Peterson, do you have the records of Brant, Tanner, and Morgan?"

Captain Peterson said, "Of course, sir," and disappeared into the outer office. He reappeared a moment later and laid three file folders on Hartfield's desk.

Hartfield never seemed to be in a hurry, and this occasion was no different. He took his time reviewing each file. The room remained dead silent, watching the Commander slowly turn and read page after page.

Wonder what would be on my file? "Sent to Hartfield Academy for breaking a boy's arm and stealing his father's car?" *That might not play so well with someone like Hartfield.*

"All three of these cadets have been here since first year. None of them have any black marks or honor issues." Hartfield sighed, tapping one finger against the top file. "I don't like to delay decisions like this, but I need to contemplate what is right. Cadets Hollister and Davidner, I will see you back here at oh-eight-hundred."

Outside Hartfield's office, Michael put a hand on Dominick's arm, looked meaningfully at him, and raised his eyebrows.

Dominick met Michael's eyes and shook his head resolutely. "Nope. It's a setup."

"Right. I don't get it. The Academy preaches honor, honor, honor. So, why risk so much for so little gain?"

"I have no idea. It doesn't make sense."

Back at the Turtle's barracks Brant had made himself scarce. The room had come back to life since Dominick and Michael had left. As soon as they walked back in, everyone gathered around them.

"So, what's up? Are they building a statue of us out front or something?" Will asked.

"It's not good, guys," Michael said. "The Badgers are accusing us of cheating. They say we stole their strategy essay."

The barrack exploded in indignant questions and cries of "Come on!" and "No way!"

"We didn't need their stupid strategy," Will said. "You had it all figured out, Michael."

Michael held his hand up to quiet them down. "There's nothing we can do about it now. We told them the truth. We didn't cheat. It's up to Hartfield now. He'll either believe us or he won't. Either way, we know we didn't do anything wrong. We know we won fair and square. That might have to be enough."

After lights out, Dominick could hear Michael tossing and turning on the bunk below him, but relaxed and laid back with his hands under his head.

We told the truth. We didn't do anything wrong. Everything will be okay.

Two minutes later, he was fast asleep.

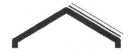

Chapter Twenty-Three

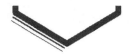

Michael and Dominick decided to skip breakfast the next day. They were standing outside Peterson's office when he arrived at 7:45. Peterson unlocked the door and let the boys into his office, which served as the outer office for Commander Hartfield. Fifteen minutes later, Peterson opened the door to Hartfield's office. He was already sitting behind his desk.

Holy crap. Does he live in here? Have like a secret Bat entrance? Slide down a fire pole?

"Cadet Davidner. Refresh my memory. How was it that you came to be with us here at the Academy?"

Oh. Okay. I can see which way this is going to go.

"I stole my dad's car and crashed it into our neighbor's shed."

Hartfield nodded. "This car of your father's—did you have his keys?"

"No sir."

"How did you manage to start the car, then?"

"I hotwired it."

"Hotwired it." Hartfield's mouth twitched. "Nine years old, unable to see over the steering wheel and reach the gas pedal at the same time, but you knew how to hotwire a car. Is that correct?"

"Yes, sir."

"How did you gain this unusual skill so early in life?"

Dominick shrugged. "I guess it's just part of what we learned in the neighborhood."

"I see. Does this neighborhood education extend to an ability to pick locks at a young age, as well?"

Dominick held Hartfield's eyes for a long moment, then broke off and looked back out the window.

"Yes, sir, but—"

"Peterson," Hartfield called, interrupting Dominick in mid-sentence.

"Yes, sir?"

"Where do you keep the strategy reports that the boys turn in ahead of the Game?"

"Locked up in my desk drawer, sir."

"And the outer office door is always locked when you're not here, is that correct?"

"Of course, sir."

"Thank you, Peterson."

"If I asked you to, could you pick the lock and gain entry to Peterson's office?"

"Yes, sir, probably, but I wouldn't."

Hartfield took a deep breath, held it for a long moment, and then released it.

"All things considered, including the testimony of three senior boys, the strategy guide being found in your barrack, and given your abilities in the arcane world of picking locks and hotwiring cars, I have no choice but to rule in the Badger's favor and declare them the winner of yesterday's Hartfield Game."

Considering all facts in evidence, you have made a mistake, sir.

"Michael, you can head off to class. Dominick, you stay here."

Michael snapped off a salute to Hartfield, laid a hand on Dominick's shoulder and quietly said, "See you in class, Dom."

As soon as Michael was gone, Hartfield said, "I spoke to your father this morning. He's on his way here to pick you up right now."

You old fraud. You already had your mind made up, so what was with the inquisition this morning?

"Lieutenant Brant has retrieved your suitcase from storage. I think it would be best if you packed your bag right now, while the rest of the Turtles are in class. Once you're packed, you can wait for your father in the library."

Dominick stood. *No need for a salute. I'm no longer a cadet.* "Commander Hartfield?"

"Yes, son?"

"You've made a mistake. I hope you figure it out eventually. A lot of good came out of my time here at the Academy. I learned a lot. I hate leaving on such a sour note."

Hartfield's eyes narrowed. "If there's more truth to be discovered, I believe we will find it."

"Thank you, sir." Dominick let himself out.

Dominick took a last tour of Hartfield Academy. He walked past the buildings, onto the track where he had run laps for making Lt. Pusser so mad. He stood at the edge of the cliff and looked out over the wild Pacific a hundred feet below.

He was surprised to find tears running down his face. *Goddamn it, I hate this. We did everything right, and we get screwed over.* He took a deep, shuddering breath and held it. *Nothing for it, though. Sometimes life just isn't fair, and that's the way it is.* He turned his back to the ocean and took in the solid, brick buildings of Hartfield Academy. *Gonna miss this place, though. Mostly the friends I made here. Two years ago, if someone had told me I would miss seeing a bunch of twelve year old kids, I would have said they were crazy. There's something about going through this process, though, that creates brothers. I really am gonna miss those guys.*

Dominick wiped his eyes and made his way to the Turtles barrack. His duffel bag sat on top of the footlocker at the very back. He looked down and realized that he was still wearing his uniform.

No need for that any more.

He quickly changed into his civilian clothes, threw his socks, underwear, and toiletries into the duffel, and laid the uniform across his bunk.

Two and a half years here, and I can pack in sixty seconds. Is that good or bad?

The clock said it was only 8:55.

Should I hang out here, and say goodbye to the Turtles? He looked around at the neat rows of footlockers and metal bunk beds. *Nah. I don't think so.*

He slung his duffel over his shoulder, walked back to the main building and sat down in the library, prepared for a long wait.

Shortly after 2:00, Joe Davidner pulled up in his old Ford. Dominick took one last look around, and hustled out to meet him. By the time the Ford pulled to a stop, Dominick was waiting for him. He opened the door and climbed in. Joe's face was twisted in a knot of anger.

Uh oh. I should have figured on this.

"Dad, I'm sorry—"

"One question, Dominick, and be sure to tell me the truth. Did you cheat?"

"No, sir."

Joe stared into his eyes for several long seconds, employing the unerring lie detector that many parents have. He nodded. "That's what I thought."

"Then why are you so mad?"

Joe's face softened. He cupped the back of Dominick's neck and pulled him to him, kissing the top of his head.

"I'm not mad at you, Nicky." He glanced furiously at the main building, where Hartfield's office was. "I hate it when people make judgements about us based on our bank accounts. If we came from a snobby neighborhood, and I earned $30,000 a year, they would have dug a little deeper, and maybe found out what the truth is."

Dominick's throat grew thick again. *Damn, it's good to be believed.*

"I love you, Dad."

"Love you too, Nicky." Joe Davidner let go of his son, and found a small smile. "I think it's for the best, anyway. I know you liked it here, but your mother and I have been wishing you were home, where you belong."

I'm not sure where I belong, Dad, other than with Emily, and I can't make that happen yet.

They pulled into the driveway back in Emeryville a little after 9:00.

Joe massaged his neck, and said, "One thing's for sure. I won't miss making that drive."

"Thanks for coming to pick me up, Dad. Sorry you had to take a day off of work."

"Forget about it. Let's go inside and see if your mom managed to keep a plate of food away from Sam."

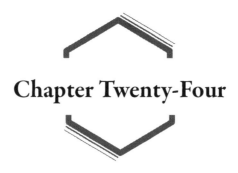

Chapter Twenty-Four

There were adjustments in getting used to civilian life for Dominick. Seven days a week, his eyes flew open and his feet hit the floor at 6:00 AM. He had become accustomed to having every minute of his day scheduled. Where finding time to just be a kid was a challenge. More than anything, though, he missed the camaraderie he'd had with Michael, Will, and the rest of the Turtles.

But, starting the school year in the middle, and having been away more than two years, at least he wasn't expected to remember where everything was. Vinny had moved away the summer before, but Wardell was still there, so he had someone to act as a guide for him.

Dominick had only been at the school for a few weeks when Christmas break arrived. By then, life had settled back into its normal rhythm, and Hartfield Academy had already begun to fade in his memory.

On New Year's Eve, Joe and Laura decided to take the kids to a movie as a special treat. They went to see *The Aristocats*, which Dominick couldn't remember seeing before.

I would have rather seen Gimme Shelter, but hey, don't look the gift parents in the mouth.

As they walked back into the house after the movie, the phone started to ring. Joe looked at his watch, then exchanged a glance with Laura.

"Who in the world would call us this late?" Laura asked. She was the first in the door, and ran to the kitchen. She picked the phone up on the seventh ring.

Nice to have a clear conscience. I haven't been in any fights, and haven't stolen any cars. Maybe it's Sam's turn to be the juvenile delinquent in the family.

"Hello?" Laura said. Then, "Yes. Just a moment, please. Joe, it's for you"

Joe handed Connie off to Laura, and picked up the receiver. "Yes?"

There was silence in the kitchen for a long time, punctuated only by Joe's, "Mmm-hmm" or "I see." Finally he said, "Thank you, Mr. Hartfield, but we are going to decline. We are moving out of state, as I've taken a job in New Mexico."

Laura raised her eyebrows at Joe, who looked at her, smiled a little, and gave a quick shake of his head, along with a guilty shrug at the lie.

"Thank you. I understand that, but no. We'll be keeping Dominick right here now. Goodbye."

Dominick stood beside his mother. "Was that about me?"

Joe sat down at the kitchen table and ran his hands through his hair. "Yes, it was. That was Hartfield. He said he owed you an apology. Apparently, one of the boys who lied about you came clean and was expelled."

Dominick nodded. "I knew it!" He said hotly. "I knew it would come out eventually. So, can I go back now?"

Joe and Laura exchanged a glance. "Nicky, your mother and I talked about this. Even if they want you to go back, we don't want you to go."

"Why not?"

"Because we think you belong here with us. The only reason we let you go there in the first place was because we didn't know what else to do."

"You just didn't want to pay my tuition," Dominick said, and regretted it immediately.

Joe winced. "Nicky, you know that's not true. If we thought it was best for you, we would have done anything to make it happen. Hartfield offered free tuition for the rest of the year as an apology. It's not about the money. It's about us wanting to be a real family again."

"So I don't get a vote, is that right?"

"I'm afraid that's right. Your mother and I have to decide what's best for you."

"Ugh!" Dominick said in frustration. He turned and stomped down the hall to the bedroom he once again shared with Sam.

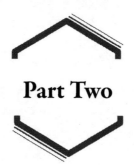

Part Two

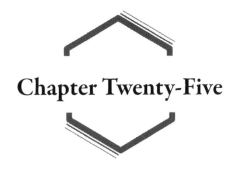

Chapter Twenty-Five

Carrie watched Dominick storm off to his room in a rage.
There's something about being in a child's body, with all the restrictions of being a child that makes people act like a child, no matter how old they really are.

She spun her pyxis clockwise and watched hours blend into days, into months, into years. The more she worked with it, the more it had become part of her. She saw the normal array of events—happy and sad, boring and exciting. She saw nothing horrible for him in the next few years, but she still worried about him.

He's not as social any more. More withdrawn than he was at the military school. She stopped for a moment and searched her memory. *And he never notices the girls who are noticing him. He loves Emily, and doesn't have eyes for anyone else. There's something about her that no one else has, at least in his eyes.*

"He loves her, whoever "she" is, and that's the end of it. When love is the answer, it doesn't matter what the question was."

Carrie jumped guiltily. She had let her mind wander and wasn't using the pyxis for its intended use—to feed the Machine.

"Hello, Bertellia. Nice to see you're back."

"Filled with a new training regimen, the more to torture you with. I notice that you were scanning ahead in that person's life. Perfectly within the rules of your pyxis, but not one of the standard techniques used. May I ask why you were scanning his path ahead?"

Because I get bored just scooping up emotions? Because I can't watch these people's lives without coming to love them?

"I admit, I come to care about the people I look over. So I look ahead to see what will befall them.

"And if something 'bad' - by your definition - is going to happen to them, what do you do then?"

"It depends. Bad things happen in everyone's lives, but if you broaden your perspective, it can turn out to be good. Say someone really wants to get a job promotion, and they miss out on it. That feels like a bad thing to them, but maybe that job would have been terrible for them in the long run, so missing out on it was really a good thing. That's why I like to look ahead for years in their life and see how things might play out."

"That's very good. That's a lesson I've been trying to reach you with for some time—perspective is everything. But, what do you do if you see something bad that, in your opinion, will continue to impact that person in a 'bad' way?"

Carrie glanced away, avoiding Bertellia's eyes. She remembered altering the scene where Dominick ran over the old man across the street. *Do I have to answer that question?*

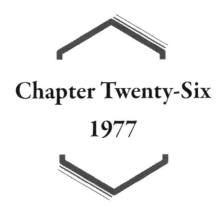

Chapter Twenty-Six
1977

Seven and a half years had passed since Dominick had returned home from Hartfield Academy. The seventies proved not to be as turbulent as the sixties had been, but still, there was Watergate, the resignation of a President, the end of the Viet Nam War, not to mention the surging popularity of disco.

Dominick already knew that his second life would not necessarily mirror his first. After all, he hadn't spent several years in a military academy the first time around. Also, in his first life, his father had developed esophageal cancer in 1975. Despite a number of surgeries, Joe Davidner had died in November 1979.

In this second life, Joe hadn't developed the cancer.

Dominick stood in the middle of the bedroom he still shared with Sam, reflecting on his current life while getting dressed.

If I have to live my whole life over just to give Dad a chance at a longer life, that's worth it. Until I factor Emily into the equation. I can't help but wonder if she is still alive somewhere, somehow, grieving me, or cursing my name for doing what I always have done—acting without thinking. Or, is Emily here, too, living out her girlhood in Wisconsin, never having heard of me. Or both? There's a reason I was an English major, not a theoretical physicist.

The boys had outgrown the bunk beds, so now the tiny room had two twin beds stuffed into the corners. Sam had graduated two years before, but had gone on to a trade school, and was now working as an apprentice electrician, a job Joe had managed to snare for him. He was earning money, but had showed no interest in leaving his mother's cooking and laundry service. Still, he was ahead of where he had been in Dominick's first life, when he had drifted from one minimum wage job to another, never finding an anchor.

Dominick slipped a tan turtleneck over his head, then picked the brown sports coat off the bed. *I've gotten used to not having my cell phone or a computer, but these seventies fashions still knock me for a loop sometimes.*

"Nicky, are you ready?" Laura called from the hallway. "We want to get there before all the parking spots are gone."

"You know I can go on my own, Mom. I do have my own car, you know."

"We are not letting you go alone to your own Baccalaureate."

"Okay, Mom. I'm almost ready." Dominick slipped on his brown loafers—*picking from all ends of the brown color spectrum today*—and grabbed a brush off the dresser. He looked in the mirror, started to pull the brush through his tangle of curls, but quickly gave up. He had let his hair grow out in the years since leaving Hartfield Academy.

He still thought often of the friends he had made there, but he hadn't been in contact with any of them. A month earlier, an envelope had arrived addressed to him, with "Please Forward" written above the address. It had been from Michael Hollister.

Hey Dom.

It was so weird having you just up and disappear that day. All this time later, we still talk about the way you stood up to Pusser to protect Will, and how you tried to take all the punishments for us for dyeing his underwear red. I still wonder what in the world we were trying to accomplish there, exactly?

I know we haven't talked since you left, but I wanted you to know that the Turtles are graduating next month, on June 7th. Most of us made it to the end. 16 Turtles will be unleashed on the world to wreak havoc. We'd love it if you could make it here.

I don't know if this letter will even reach you, but if it does, you need to know that being a Turtle is something that neither time, nor soap and a good scrubbing, can wash away. You're with us for life – whether you like it or not.

Michael

Dominick toyed with the idea of driving up and attending. He knew the rest of the guys would be glad to see him, and he did have his own car—a '67 Chevelle Super Sport that would have been the envy of all his middle-aged friends in 1999—and his own graduation would be over by then.

Dominick set the hairbrush down, gave himself one last inspection in the mirror, and hustled off to his Baccalaureate.

AFTER HIS GRADUATION from Emeryville High, Dominick decided to make the drive north and attend the Hartfield Academy graduation. At dinner that night, when he told his parents that he was driving up for the ceremony, they weren't exactly enthusiastic.

"I understand you think it would be nice to see your friends, but you haven't seen or spoken to them in years," Joe said.

"Will you even have anything in common with them, now?" Laura chimed in.

"Besides," Joe said, picking up the attack, "what did Hartfield Academy ever do for you?"

"They taught me a lot, Dad. They gave me a lot of discipline, and going there was good for me. Maybe you guys have forgotten what I was like, why you sent me there. Have I gotten into any trouble since I got back?"

Both Joe and Laura shook their heads.

Before they could speak, Dominick continued, "I know I haven't seen them in a long time, but when we were young, we formed a bond. I think I need to bring it full circle. For closure, if nothing else."

Two days later, Dominick got up at 5:00 AM, and was on the road by 5:30. The completion of Interstate 5 in the intervening years would have made for a faster drive, but Dominick took the old route, just for nostalgia's sake.

The graduation was scheduled for 2:00 PM, and Dominick pulled his Chevelle onto the Hartfield driveway half an hour before that. As he drove around the circular drive, he noted a headstone neatly sitting between the two flagpoles. *Wonder when they started burying people here on the Academy grounds? Did Hartfield kick the bucket or something?*

He found a parking spot at the back of the overflow parking lot and walked over to where the ceremony was being held. A stage had been set up at the back of the lawn, with folding chairs in front, and temporary bleachers built on each side. The chairs were mostly empty, but the bleachers were filling up quickly. Dominick slipped into a spot at the back and sat down. No one had recognized him.

Soon, the Turtles filed in and took their seats at the front of the stage.

The graduation began right on time. *I would have expected nothing less.*

Commander Hartfield, a little older, grayer, and looking much thinner than Dominick remembered him, stepped to the podium and made his welcoming remarks.

He looks like he's aged twenty years.

"Good afternoon, cadets, parents and loved ones, and of course, Turtles."

"Welcome to another graduation ceremony at Hartfield Academy. This is always a proud, yet sad moment. Over the last decade, I've had the privilege of watching these boys grow and mature, to become splendid young men, and wonderful examples of the brotherhood we hope will develop with each new class. Every class is special, of course, but the Turtles are unique. In the entire history of the Academy, they are the only class to ever win the Hartfield Game the first year they played."

A cheer erupted from the Turtles, along with smiles and pats on the back.

Nice to hear our honor has been restored.

"Enough from me, though. Before we begin handing out diplomas, I'd like to bring up our valedictorian, Will Summer. Will?"

A tall, sandy-haired boy in an immaculate dress uniform stood straight and tall and stepped up to the microphone.

Holy heck, maybe Mom and Dad were right. I don't think I'd have recognized Will. He grew up a lot. Dominick lifted up off his seat an inch or two and craned his neck to see if he could spot Michael, too, but he was lost in the sea of Turtles.

"Thank you, Commander Hartfield, and thank you to the Hartfield Academy instructors and staff who have put up with us all these years. I suppose I should also apologize to Lieutenant Pusser and the string of prefects who followed him for all the terrible things we did to them." He looked back at the Turtles with a huge smile.

The Turtles cheered. A squat, heavyset man in his late twenties, dressed in a US Army uniform and sitting a few rows in front of Dominick stood and waved in acknowledgment.

That's gotta be him. Hello, Pusser. Dominick smiled to himself at the thought of the many ways they had tortured him.

"Seriously, though, every Turtle and every instructor knows that I'm not who should be standing up here, representing our class. Michael Hollister should be."

Dominick craned his neck again and saw a blond crew cut in the front row shaking back and forth.

"Michael was so far ahead of us, he ended up teaching us almost as much as our instructors did. When we were just scared, homesick First Years, Michael was the calming force that held the Turtles together. The only reason I'm up here instead of Michael is because that's the way he wanted it. And that says a lot about him too, doesn't it? Every Turtle could stand up here and tell a story of how Michael helped them out, but we don't have that much time, so here's mine. There used to be a tradition at Hartfield that if you wet your bed, you had to carry your sheets with you all day as a public humiliation."

Dominick's eyes glazed over as he became lost in the memory of that early day in the barracks where he and a few others had stood up for Will.

"I was the first Turtle to do so, and I was assigned to carry my soaking sheets around the grounds that day. First, Dominick Davidner, our brother who is not here, stood up for me; then Michael peed on his own sheets and carried them with him, so I wouldn't be alone."

Dominick jumped a little at hearing his own name. *They haven't forgotten me.*

"Think about that for a minute," Will continued. "How easy is it to stand by and watch someone else be punished when you are innocent? How difficult is it to put yourself in the line of fire? That's what Michael did for me, and I know he did things just like that for every single Turtle. He did that nine years ago. I'll never forget it."

Will took one step back from the podium and, in a voice that carried to every corner of the Academy, said, "Turtles! Attention!" All the Turtles jumped to attention. They all faced Michael. "Salute."

Without a thought, Dominick stood in place and snapped off a perfect salute toward Michael, as well. A few people in the crowd turned to look at him, but none of the Turtles saw him.

With his back to the rest of the audience, Michael stood and saluted back.

Applause broke out throughout the crowd.

Dominick sat back down, surprised to find a lump in his throat and his eyes wet.

Before the applause died down, Will walked back to his seat and Hartfield began calling out names to come and accept their diplomas. It took Dominick a few names to adjust to the new reality in front of him. Twelve year old boys had suddenly transformed into eighteen-year-old young men—but he got the hang of it and started recognizing Turtles before their names were called.

Hartfield Academy did its job. It turned this group of boys into men, and now they are ready to be soldiers, if they want to be.

Once the ceremony was complete, the crowd broke up into smaller groups, each celebrating their own graduate. Dominick spotted Michael, standing off by himself, watching the proceedings.

Dominick walked over and stood right in front of him, a small smile on his lips. "Hello, Genius."

Michael's mouth fell slightly open and his eyebrows shot up. "Dom? Dominick, is that you?"

Dominick nodded, his smile growing. Michael opened his arms and embraced him.

Pretty different for the kid that didn't like to be touched by anybody.

"I'm so glad you made it. The guys will be really happy to see you. It didn't feel right doing this without you. So, how are you?"

"All is good. Graduated from high school last week, set free on the world now."

Michael shook his head. "Damnit, you should have been here with us today. Hey, did you drive all the way up from New Mexico?

Commander Hartfield said that was part of the reason you couldn't come back, because you were moving."

"No, that was just something my Dad made up, because he was pissed at Hartfield. He just wouldn't let me come back. I think the whole thing hurt his pride. I wanted to come back, but they wouldn't let me."

Michael shook his head. "What a waste. It would have been so great to have you here all this time." He put his arm around Dominick's shoulder and said, "Come on, the rest of the guys are going to flip when they see you."

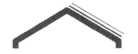

Chapter Twenty-Seven

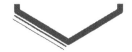

Bertella reached out and touched Carrie's Pyxis. "Well?"

"What do I do, if I think things are going to turn out disastrously for them?"

"That was my question, yes," Bertellia said, patiently.

Might as well bite the bullet. She never asks a question she doesn't already know the answer to, anyway.

"I help them."

Bertella's serene expression didn't change. "How exactly do you help them?"

"I ... move time back and forth. Give them a chance to do things slightly differently."

"Does that work? Does it present the desired result for you?"

"Sometimes."

"And when it doesn't?"

In for a penny ...

"I pull strands of the image away and manipulate what happens, until it turns out better for everyone." Carrie paused, then rushed on, "I don't ever do it if it's going to hurt someone else. That's not fair." She realized she had used that word—*fair*—and winced.

"How did you learn how to do this? To manipulate events like this?"

"I don't know. It just seemed natural. Doesn't everyone do that?"

"Have you seen anyone else doing that?"

"Well, no, but I don't think they saw me do it either."

"Perhaps they didn't, but here, someone is always watching."

"Are you forbidding me to do this? To help my people?"

Bertellia smiled at Carrie's use of the phrase "my people." "'Forbid' is such a strong word. No, I never forbid anything. However, I can tell you that it will be better for you if you stop doing this, and simply focus on feeding the Machine."

"Better for me?" Carrie laughed, and there was a bitter, ironic tone to it. "What can be done to me? As you have said, I am perfect, and invulnerable. I cannot ever be truly hurt."

"True enough. You cannot. Your circumstances can be changed, though, so that life itself feels painful."

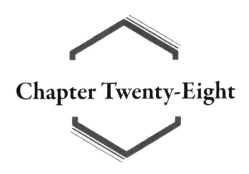

Chapter Twenty-Eight

Joe and Laura wanted Dominick to keep *Davidner and Son Small Engine Repair* going over the summer, to help him with his college tuition, but Dominick had other plans. After waiting through what felt like the eternity of ten years, Dominick knew it was finally the right time to go and find Emily.

He had actually enjoyed being in high school again, as he allowed himself to excel enough to get into the Honors program, which brought him more challenging work. It also looked good on his school record which, along with his 3.90 grade point average, would allow him to get into any college in the region shy of Stanford. The problem was, he didn't want to go.

Once I've found Emily, and we're together again, then it will feel right to think about college, and our future. But I can't focus on anything but her until I find her.

Dominick's initial plan was to take the money he had saved from repairing engines and head for the Midwest as soon as possible. The day after graduation, once again eating hamburger hash with the entire family, Dominick broke the idea of leaving.

"So, I know you guys want me to head off to college in the fall—"

"—With those grades, you better," Joe interrupted.

"—but, I don't think I'm quite ready."

"Oh, no, none of this, 'I'm gonna go backpack around Europe and find myself' nonsense for you, Nicky. You're going to school. You've worked too hard to give this up."

Dominick bit his lip. He had anticipated resistance, but not quite this strong.

"Listen, Dad, I'm not saying I don't want to go to college. I do. I just want to go see the country first. Other than one trip to Idaho to see Uncle Frank two summers ago, I haven't seen anything yet."

"There's plenty of time for that later."

"But there isn't, not really. Think about it, Dad. First I'm in college, then fall in love, and then I've got a job and I'll have a couple of rugrats of my own to support. Maybe, if I'm lucky, two weeks of vacation every year. And, those two weeks are probably spent putting up a new fence, or painting the house, just like you did."

Joe put his fork down and looked at Laura first, then back at Dominick. He said quietly, "That's not such a bad life." He swept his hand around the table, at Sam, still in his work overalls, Connie, just turned thirteen, and wearing braces, and Dominick himself. "It hasn't been the most exciting life in the world, but it's been a rewarding one all the same."

Dominick dropped his head. *I didn't mean to denigrate what you did, or how you lived your life, Dad.*

He looked up and made eye contact with Joe and then his mother. "I love you, Dad, Mom. I am thankful for what you've done for me. For all of us. I know you only want what's best for me, and I appreciate your perspective. But, I'm going to do this. I'm going to go out into the world and see what's out there."

And see where Emily is.

Joe nodded. "Well, I can't stop you, I suppose. But..."

There's always a 'but', isn't there?

"Have you looked at our shop out there? Have you seen all the lawn mowers, boat engines, and rototillers lined up alongside and behind the shed? There's a few month's work out there, even if we're both working on them. If I have to do them all by myself ..." Joe let the thought hang in the air.

I know when I'm beaten. It's just check, though, Dad, not checkmate.

"You're right. It's not fair for me to just take off and leave you with all that work." Dominick pushed his food around. "How about this, then? How about if we work on all those motors together until they're all done, but we stop accepting new work? Is that fair?"

"That's fair," Joe said, and took a long pull on his Budweiser. "I don't like it, but it's fair."

DOMINICK ESTIMATED that if he really applied himself, he could wade through the backload of small engines in two or three weeks, a month tops, then he could be on his way. What he failed to count in his estimation was his own ability to say 'No.'"

It started the very next morning. Joe was at work, but Dominick got up early and took down the small sign out front that read "Davidner and Son." He had gone straight to fixing Mr. Hansen's mower. Very few of the jobs were challenging, just time-consuming, if he wanted to do them right. He was rolling the mower out to the front of the yard where Mr. Hansen could collect it that afternoon, when Mr. Bratski appeared from across the street, pushing the same old mower that Joe and Dominick had been fixing for six years.

"It's been a year, young Dominick. Time to tune her up. She never runs as good as that first day you bring her back."

"Oh, I'm sorry, Mr. Bratski. I'm getting ready to leave town, so we're not taking any more jobs. I'm just trying to finish up with the ones we've got."

Mr. Bratski muttered, "Oh, I see." Then he sucked on his false teeth and looked pained. "I don't have a truck. I don't even know how I can get the mower to those thieves at Wilson's repair." More teeth sucking. "I hate to pay what they charge, after doing business with you all these years. I think I was your very first customer, wasn't I?"

Dominick knew when he was being hustled, but he still couldn't take it. "Okay, okay, leave it here. I'll get it tuned up for you. But, please promise me, you won't tell anyone."

"Not a word," Mr. Bratski promised.

Later that afternoon, widowed Mrs. Lemkins appeared in the shadow of the garage door. "Mr. Bratski tells me that I had better get this old mower over to you pronto, because you're closing up shop soon."

Dominick again recognized he was beaten. "Just put it there next to Mr. Bratski's, Mrs. Lemkins. I'll get to it as soon as I can."

The fact that he wouldn't accept any more business was the best advertising he could have done. Everyone wanted to take advantage of quality work at cheap prices.

That night, after supper, Dominick went back out to the shop to try to get ahead of the backlog. Shortly after he tore into a mower, Joe wandered into the shop. "Need any help with that?"

Things had been tense since Dominick had announced he was leaving, and not planning on going on to college right away. Dominick shook his head. "Nah, I've got this, Dad." He looked up from the carburetor he was working on. Joe stood in the doorway with his back to him, looking out into the setting sun.

"But," Dominick said, "I do have that Evinrude motor torn apart and I was having a hard time figuring out what the problem was. Would you mind looking it over for me?"

Joe turned and looked at Dominick and smiled.

He knows that's bullshit, but it doesn't matter. It's the way men are.

"Sure, I'll take a look at it, see what I can see." He sauntered over to the engine and looked down his nose at it, poking here and there. He began to whistle along to the old country song playing softly on the radio hanging on a nail in the corner.

Just like that, the summer melted away—Dominick working and sweating alone during the daytime, but sharing long hours with his Dad at night. They both knew they were on the cusp of a major sea change in their life. They also both recognized that this experience, working elbow to elbow, cussing a little and laughing a lot, was one that would likely never be repeated.

Eventually, September rolled around and the flow of repair jobs slowed, then stopped altogether.

Good thing we don't live in the mountains, or the snowmobile repair jobs would start, and I'd never get out of here.

On September 3rd, Joe and Dominick both finished off the last jobs they had, and looked around the bare shop. They cleaned and put away their tools. *A place for everything and everything in its place* was Joe's lifelong motto, and he had passed it on to Dominick. As Dominick was putting away the last of the tools, Joe said, "Just a minute," and walked out of the garage.

He reappeared a few minutes later, with two cans of Budweiser. "Probably won't make your mother very happy, but I think it's called for." He handed one to Dominick and popped the tab on the other. "I know you've been itching to get out of here for months now, but you stuck around and did the right thing. The world needs more people who are willing to put off what they want in order to do what's right. I'm proud of you."

Dominick's eyes glistened. He looked down at the can of beer so his dad wouldn't see the tears. He opened his can and took a tentative swallow.

Been more than ten years since I've had a beer. It's still good.

"Thanks, Dad. I … I think I'm gonna get packed up and take off tomorrow."

"I know," was all Joe said.

They drank the rest of their beers in silence, then went into the house.

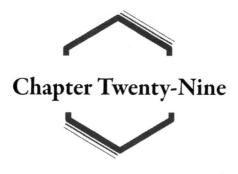

Chapter Twenty-Nine

When Dominick set about packing the next morning, he realized that he had carried over at least some of the habits he had picked up at Hartfield Academy, in that he still didn't like to have too many possessions. He had enough clothes to fill his duffel, and he packed his essential tools into the tool box his parents had bought him the previous Christmas, but there wasn't much else he felt compelled to take.

When Joe had told Laura that Dominick was leaving the next morning, she had bustled around the kitchen making him a care package of food—meatloaf sandwiches, Tupperware with leftover lasagna, half a loaf of homemade bread—to get him through the first few days on the road.

Dominick was up early and had a chance to say goodbye to both Laura and Joe before they left for work. Joe's goodbye was quick—a wave, a nod, and a "be good, son" as he hurried out the door.

Laura would have none of that. She held him close for a long minute, then reached up to hold his face in both her hands, turning it from side to side, memorizing who he was at that moment. Finally, she laid her head against his chest, listening to his heartbeat. She said, simply, "I love you, Nicky," then turned and hurried out the door.

Dominick turned to see that Connie, now a beautiful young woman, and a freshman in high school, was standing behind him, watching the goodbyes and laughing a little.

"Do they think you're dying? You're just going for a drive, right?"

"Right. I think it's just that Sam hasn't left home yet—"

"And I don't think he ever will, as long as Mom is feeding him."

"—so this is the first time they've seen one of their kids leave home. Even when I went to Hartfield, they knew where I was and that they could get me at any time. I understand it. Listen, I'm probably going to be gone for a while, but I'll call home every week. So, if you need to talk, we can."

"Thanks, big brother."

"No 'Bubby' anymore?"

"Fine. Thanks, Bubby." She rolled her eyes, but Dominick could still see her eyes glistened.

"Okay, gonna take off."

"Where are you staying tonight?"

"No idea. Ain't it great?"

"I'm fine with staying in my comfy bed, thanks."

Dominick opened the front door, stepped to the edge of the small porch, and felt an exultation he had never felt before. He leaped off the top step, over the tiny border of flowers, and onto the lawn. He slid in behind the wheel of the Chevelle and turned her over.

The deep purr of the V8 engine, so much power ready to be unleashed at a moment's notice, thrilled Dominick as it always did. He smiled to himself and turned the radio on.

Gotta have some tunes for a momentous occasion like this.

"*Don't Give Up On Us, Baby*" by David Soul, was playing.

Nope. Not quite right.

He pushed a button on the radio, and a generic rock 'n roll song came on. The DJ back-announced, "That's a moldy oldie you don't hear much anymore, if you ever did—*Rock 'n Roll Boogaloo*, by Jimmy Velvet and the Black Velvets. Now, here's the Righteous Brothers, and *Rock 'n Roll Heaven*."

Dominick pushed another button and tuned in 680 KFRC, out of San Francisco. "Feels Like the First Time," by Foreigner came through the speakers. He listened for a moment, nodding his head, tapping his fingers against the steering wheel.

I've been planning, thinking about, and waiting for this moment to arrive for more than ten years. Now that it's finally here, I feel a little nervous. Is she really out there? What will she say, when she sees me? Will she recognize me in any way, on any level?

He turned up the driving guitar line of "Feels Like the First Time," slipped the car into reverse, and backed out of the driveway. The bump at the edge of the driveway always made him think of stealing his father's Dodge and wreaking havoc on Mr. Bratski's rose bushes and shed. On this day, he manage to pull onto the street without incident.

As he pulled out, he saw Mr. Bratski, a little rounder and a little shorter than he had been on that day ten years earlier, standing out in the yard in his dark socks that went up to his knees, and his yellow shorts pulled up past his navel, with the newspaper tucked under one arm, and a cup of coffee in his hand. He waved.

Dominick smiled and waved back, but resisted the urge to give a jaunty honk of the horn—it was still early, and wouldn't be appreciated in their quiet little neighborhood—and tooled on down the street.

Toward the freeway.

Toward freedom.

Finally, toward Emily.

Chapter Thirty

Dominick had bought a AAA Road Atlas the year before, and had been studying it ever since. The easiest trip for him would have been to get on Interstate 80 in Emeryville and stay on it almost all the way to Sheboygan, Wisconsin. In another few years, he would have been able to have taken that epic freeway all the way, but in 1977, there were a few areas where construction wasn't completed.

No matter. Dominick wasn't interested in driving 2,300 miles of freeway, anyway. In fifty-one years of living, he'd never had much of a chance to travel. In his first life, he had graduated high school and gone straight to college. After graduating, he had taken a job teaching high school English in an inner city school in Oakland. After a few years there, he had accepted a position in Middle Falls, Oregon, which seemed like a slice of heaven after working in a school where drugs and violence had been an everyday occurrence. Middle Falls remained heavenly until he learned in the most abrupt fashion possible that violence wasn't just for inner city schools anymore.

Once he met and fell in love with Emily, they never had money to travel. They had summers off, yes, but two teachers' salaries never got them far. Many summers, the house needed a major repair so they fixed the house and often ended up taking other jobs in the summer to make ends meet.

In any case, he had never traveled. Now he was a fifty-one year old man in a fit, healthy, eighteen year old body. He had a tuned up '67 Chevelle Super Sport, and he had $800 in his pockets. Not a fortune, but in 1977, gas was sixty cents a gallon, and if you didn't care too much about amenities, you could find a roadside motel for eight bucks. The road, and his second life, stretched out in front of him, filled with endless possibilities.

If he had wanted, Dominick could have made the drive to Wisconsin in two days. Instead, he took a week. He drifted north first, hugging the California coast wherever possible. By mid-afternoon, he rolled through Crescent City. A few miles later, he saw the driveway that led to Hartfield Academy. He contemplated turning in to say hello.

Ah, mid-September. Michael and everyone I ever knew there, other than the instructors, are gone. I don't need to just look at the buildings again.

He pushed on north. He spent the first night in a tiny motel called The Blue Horizon, just over the Oregon state line, in Brookings. The room was $8.50, but there was a .50 charge for towels. Dominick saved the two quarters and got by with the towel he had brought along in his duffel. It got dark earlier as fall approached, but he still got there in time to enjoy the sunset on the beach before retiring to his room for a dinner of leftover lasagna and two slices of homemade bread.

The next morning, he drove north to Newport, Oregon, then turned east to catch I-5. Less than half an hour later, he took the turnoff for Middle Falls.

The town didn't look that much different to him in 1977 than it had when he had last seen it in 1999. There had been a few more fast food options, and the Blockbuster video he had always gone to wasn't built yet, but the residential streets looked unchanged.

Without thinking, he drove to the house that he and Emily had shared. It was a small, two-bedroom brick rambler with a white picket fence and a detached single car garage. If he closed his eyes and squinted a bit, Dominick could picture himself and Emily standing in the driveway, saying goodbye on the day he was killed. He sat there for ten minutes, drinking in the nostalgia and memories.

I'll have nothing but memories, unless I start moving.

Dominick left Middle Falls behind with some regret, but turned north toward Washington. He turned east just over the Washington line, then followed the mighty Columbia River for more than a hundred miles. He crossed over into Idaho, then cut across Montana. He spent his second and third nights sleeping in the back of the Chevelle.

Maybe I should have gotten a van instead of a sports car. I wouldn't have looked as cool going down the road, but I'd sure sleep better.

On the fourth day, he dropped down into Wyoming. He'd seen an ad on the television for the upcoming movie, *Close Encounters of the Third Kind,* and that reminded him to stop and see Devils Tower. He arrived at the tower via a back road, and spotted it first from a distance. It did look odd, such a huge formation shooting up from nowhere, with nothing like it anywhere around.

Hmmm. It's cool, but once you see it, you've kind of seen it.

He spent the next night in a dingy motel in Rapid City and drove down to see Mount Rushmore the next day.

Same thing as Devils Tower. It's cool to see in person what I've only seen in pictures, but once you've looked at it for five minutes, what else is there to do? Buy a pennant or a refrigerator magnet in the gift shop? I think it's time to stop sightseeing, so I can get to Emily,

Dominick hustled to the Chevelle, drove back to Interstate 90, and headed east. He drove through the night, and just as the sun was rising, he crossed the Sheboygan city limits. He drove straight through the town until he ran into the shores of Lake Michigan.

He worked his way around the lake until he found a quiet residential area, then pulled over onto a side street. He didn't even bother to leave the driver's seat. Instead he just pulled a ball cap over his eyes, laid the seat back, and was asleep within minutes.

Less than an hour later, he was awakened by a metallic tapping on his window. He lifted the brim of the cap to see what was disturbing him and looked into the face of one of Sheboygan's finest. He was a young patrolman and he was making the universal "roll down your window" gesture.

Dominick jumped a little, startled and still groggy. He rolled down the window halfway. Chilly air rushed in.

Ah, Late September in Wisconsin can be a little chillier than the Bay Area. Guess I should have known that.

"Yes?" Dominick said, after clearing his throat.

"Can I ask what you're doing, son?"

Son, my ass. If you're more than twenty-five, I'll eat your badge.

Dominick mustered his best smile, then said, "Sleeping?"

The cop lowered his chin a bit, then sighed like a twenty year veteran. "Sheboygan has an anti-vagrancy law on the books. I'm going to ask you to move along."

Dominick smiled a little broader. "Vagrancy? That's a little harsh, isn't it? I drove all night and just pulled into town. It was too early to rent a motel room."

The police officer straightened and hitched up his gun belt. "Oh, new in town, huh? Well, that makes all the difference. I can offer you a tour of the sights. We'll start with our holding cell, then move on to a look inside one of our courtrooms. After that, you can spend a few nights learning what Sheboygan hospitality is all about at our gray bar motel."

Really? For taking a nap in my car? Okay, Barney Fife, have it your way.

"Do you have a license for operating this motor vehicle?"

Dominick sighed, chuckled a little to himself, then reached for his wallet and produced his license. He dug around in the glove compartment and found his registration, then handed it over.

The officer took the license and registration and retreated to his prowler.

Dominick stretched and rubbed the sleep out of his eyes.

This'll be a great first call home. Hey, Dad, I'm in Wisconsin. I'm under arrest for vagrancy.

A few minutes later, the officer returned to Dominick's window. "You're good to go, son, but I'd advise you to do just that: go. If I see you sleeping in one of the neighborhoods on my beat, I'll run you in."

"Which neighborhoods are on your beat?"

The young cop, puffed his chest out a little and said, "All of them. By the way, if you're planning on staying in our fair city, you'll have thirty days to change from this California license to a Wisconsin one." He dragged the syllables of *California* out so that it sounded exotic.

"Thank you, officer," Dominick said. He replaced the registration, slipped his license back in his wallet, and turned the key. He was careful not to give it much gas as he pulled away.

I'd probably violate some noise ordinance and give him another reason to run me in.

Dominick drove until he found a parking spot in the downtown area right in front of a small café with a sign out front that read, simply, "Al's."

He hopped out of the Chevelle, locked her up, and went inside. There were a few tables scattered around, plus a long bar with red barstools. Dominick took a seat at the bar and turned the heavy ceramic cup over.

Within seconds, a waitress with heavy makeup and dyed red hair appeared with a coffee pot and filled his cup.

"Know what you want?"

"Uh ..." He hadn't even seen a menu yet. "Two eggs, over easy?"

"Bacon or sausage?"

"Oh, bacon, definitely."

"Hang on, hon, it'll be up in two shakes."

"Excuse me," Dominick said, looking at her name tag, "Doris, do you have a newspaper lying around anywhere?"

"What, the Depression? Sure, hang on." She reached under the counter and pulled out a newspaper, laying it on the counter in front of him. The masthead read, "The Sheboygan Press."

I get it. Press – Depression. Everybody's a comedian.

' While he waited for his breakfast, he scanned the Help Wanted ads. Not much looked promising, but he did see one garage looking for a mechanic. *That might work.*

Dominick wolfed his breakfast down so fast, Sam would have been proud.

Doris came to check on him and saw that the plate was clean. "Didn't like it, huh? Surprised you didn't eat the plate."

Dominick smiled, stripped three singles off his bankroll and dug two quarters out of his pocket for a tip. On the way out of the café, he stopped at the payphone and pulled the Sheboygan and Surrounding Area phone book out. He flipped to the white pages until he found the names beginning with the letter E. He turned a few more pages, then ran his finger down the left-hand column until he found the name he was looking for: Harvey and Louise Esterhaus. The address said they lived at 2117 Martens Street.

With his heart nearly beating out of his chest, Dominick drove through several residential neighborhoods, hoping to stumble across Martens Street. Finally, he gave up and pulled into a Phillips 66 gas station. As the pump jockey filled his tank, Dominick asked for directions to Martens Street.

Ten minutes later, he found what he was looking for, turned onto it and followed it to the 2100 block. He missed 2117 the first time, so had to turn around in a driveway and circle back. This time, he carefully counted the houses down as he passed them. 2143, 2137, finally, there it was. A lovely two story white colonial. The lawn and hedges were neatly trimmed, and the walkways recently swept. The leaves that had started to fall in a few spots had already been raked and collected.

This would have been a lot easier if they had still lived in this house when Emily and I were married, but they had already downsized to the condo by the lake by then.

Dominick pulled to the curb just past the house. He put his hand on the door handle to get out when the front door swung open and three girls emerged. They were dressed casually in high-waisted bellbottom jeans and knit tops. The colors of their outfits were different, but managed to convey the idea that they were together. Friends.

Dominick leaned toward the passenger window so he could see more clearly. The girls on either side faded away. An electric shock ran from the top of his head, down his spine and to his toes. The girl in the middle, had long, blonde hair, a heart-shaped face, and a laugh on her lips.

Emily.

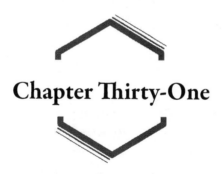

Chapter Thirty-One

Tears sprang to Dominick's eyes.

Emily. Eleven years I've waited for you. I wasn't even sure you would really be here. But, there you are, so young and beautiful, I can hardly stand it. Emily! I love you!

Once again, his hand reached for the door handle. Once again, he stopped himself.

Hold on, hold on. Keep it together. She doesn't know me from Adam. If I come on too strong, it will freak her out, and then where will I be? Trying to explain that I'm really a time traveler, and that we were already married in her future? That I'm her soul mate? Down that path, only madness lies.

Slightly slack-jawed, Dominick adjusted his mirror so he could watch the girls climb into a station wagon. Emily slid behind the wheel, looked over her shoulder and turned down the street headed the other way. Dominick shifted into drive and did a three-point turn on the narrow residential street. By the time he was pointing in the opposite direction, they were several blocks ahead.

Dominick didn't push it. It was mid-morning, and traffic was light. They got on the Interstate for a few miles, but then got right back off and headed southeast. Eventually, they passed a sign that said, "University of Wisconsin–Sheboygan."

Light dawned on Dominick. *She must be going to college here. But, that's not right. She graduated from the UW, but it was UW-Madison, not Sheboygan.* He watched the station wagon turn into a parking lot. Immediately, the three girls hopped out and, now carrying book bags, hurried, still laughing, into a building and disappeared.

Dominick tapped his fingers against the wheel. *So. Things are different here, I guess. I didn't go to Hartfield Academy for two years in my last life, either. It's the butterfly effect. Change one small thing and it causes ripples through the world.* He turned the wheel to loop a circle around the parking lot and out. *Doesn't matter, though. I saw her. I saw Emily. Everything is going to be okay now. For the first time in a very long time, everything is going to be okay.*

DOMINICK SPENT THE next hour driving around Sheboygan, getting the lay of the land, familiarizing himself with the neighborhoods. In the end, he drove back to the college—not seeking Emily, it was too early for that. But, now that he knew she was here, he knew he would be too. At least, for a while. That meant he needed some cheap housing. Wherever students were, cheap housing typically followed, so he parked outside the Student Union Building and went inside. Sure enough, just inside the entry, there was a bulletin board with different notices—ride shares, offers of tutoring, and rooms for rent. Dominick tore off several of the tags of different ads, then wandered around until he found a payphone.

He started with five possibilities, but struck out on the first four. *Maybe trying to compete for student housing right after a new semester starts isn't the smartest idea in the world.*

When he called the fifth number, a man's gruff voice answered.

"Crow's," he said.

"Excuse me?" Dominick asked, caught off-guard.

Whatever minimal patience the man seemed to possess was used up in that one question. "Crow residence," he said, enunciating slowly, as though Dominick might be slightly slow.

"Oh, yes. I see. I'm calling about the room for rent. Is it still available?"

"No, rented that last week."

"Ah. Of course. Well ..."

"I *do* have something left, if you ain't picky, though."

Dominick didn't like the sound of the man. He also didn't relish the idea of draining through his savings, staying in a motel for very many nights, either.

"Can I come see it?"

"Suit yourself. I'm always home." He rattled off an address in one of the neighborhoods Dominick had driven through earlier.

Not a bad area. Close to the college.

"I'm on my way."

Fifteen minutes later, Dominick parked on the street below a towering, slightly seedy house that was likely the bane of the neighborhood. All the other houses were well-painted and maintained. The Crow residence gutters were slightly askew, the paint was peeling, and the screen on the front door hung at an odd angle.

Nonetheless, Dominick walked up the steps to the house and knocked on the front door. A voice on the other side yelled, "Come around to the side door!"

Dominick peeked through the glass on the door to see if something might be blocking the door, but the path appeared clear.

Hmm. Odd.

He followed a small path around the side of the house, found another door, and knocked again. It seemed to take Mr. Crow a long time to arrive, especially since he knew Dominick was going to it.

Finally the door opened, and a tall, heavy, mostly bald man filled the door. He was dressed in pajamas that might have been a Christmas gift during the Eisenhower era.

"Hello, I'm Dominick Davidner. I called about a room?"

Gene Crow looked Dominick up and down. Finally, he grunted, turned away from the door and said over his shoulder, "Come on, then."

The side door led into a small porch, and then a kitchen, which was in somewhat better condition than the exterior of the house would have led him to believe. Mr. Crow shambled ahead, through the kitchen, then a dining room piled with magazines and discarded junk mail, and into a dimly lit living room. At the end of the living room, there was a large fireplace. Mr. Crow strolled over to it, turned around, and stared at Dominick. "Well, come here."

"Oh!" Dominick said, unaware that his presence was required there.

"This is the Mantle of Fame." The way he said it, Dominick could actually hear the capital letters.

Dominick leaned politely forward to examine the Mantle of Fame. There were a few dusty nick knacks, along with a series of Polaroids leaning up against them. Crow plucked the first one between his meaty fingers and said, "This is Jin Lee," he said, proudly. "He studied at the university and went on to get a doctorate in Biochemistry. He came here from his home country, all by himself, and became a doctor. Graduated third in his class."

Dominick looked politely at the photo, which showed a young Asian man, standing in front of the very same fireplace, dressed in a suit, with a broad smile on his face. *By the looks of the suit, and that horrible tie he's wearing, I'd guess mid-sixties.*

Crow replaced the photo gingerly, then picked the next one up.

Oh, my God. Dominick looked the length of the mantle, dotted with Polaroids. *Please tell me he's not going to give me a biography of every person in these damn pictures.*

He did. One at a time, he picked up each photo and recited what soon became apparent was a memorized speech about each of them. Dominick cast his eyes about, looking for any escape, but there was none. He was trapped.

Forty-five minutes later, the lecture at the Mantle of Fame was over. Dominick hesitated to speak, afraid that he might cause him to start over and go through the whole damn speech again, but he spoke up anyway. "Is it possible for me to see the room?"

Crow looked at him reproachfully, as though he had committed a serious breach in etiquette. "All in good time, my boy, all in good time. First, I will need to go over the house rules and take you through the rest of the house."

Sweet Jesus, just kill me now.

Finally, after another hour of interminable details about which shelf of the refrigerator went with which room, when acceptable TV hours were, and on and on and on, Crow folded his hands across his protruding belly and said, "I suppose you'd like to see the room now?"

"Yes, please," Dominick said with a sigh. The tour had nearly sucked his will to live but he figured he had gone this far, he may as well see the room.

"Well," Crow said, leaning in like a conspirator, "it's not one of my regular rooms, but I've been working on it the last few days. It's downstairs. He opened a door and led Dominick down an L-shaped staircase, into a dank, smelly basement. In two corners of the basement, 8 X 10 bedrooms had been sheetrocked in. In the third corner, a coin-operated washer and dryer stood, noisily working away. In the final corner, there were heavy army surplus blankets hung from rafters that reached all the way to the ground.

"I haven't gotten around to putting the drywall up, yet, but I thought this might work out fine for a single young man, if he wasn't too picky." He walked to the blankets and threw one back with a theatrical flair. "It comes furnished with a bed and nightstand. There's even a light." He said the last as though he were Ricardo Montalban, pitching "Rich Corinthian leather."

Dominick twisted up his face, but poked his head into the space. An old rug had been thrown down over the concrete floor. The walls themselves were also concrete. A bare bulb hung down in the middle of the room. To one side, a twin bed and small night stand stood forlornly. A window above the bed and about three quarters of the way up the wall showed where ground level was.

Crow smiled broadly, which did not make him any more attractive. "I charge $125 per month for everyone else, but I thought I could let this room go for, oh, maybe $110?"

Dominick chuckled a little to himself, then said, "I'll give you $60 a month."

Crow took a half step back, as if offended. He stroked his chin like a villain in a Saturday serial, then said, "Done. I'll need first, last, and a deposit against any phone calls you make."

Dominick hesitated, but eventually reached out and shook Mr. Crow's offered hand.

Chapter Thirty-Two

Dominick fought his initial urge to drive back to Emily's house and introduce himself.

Hello, I'm Dominick, your soul mate and one true love. In my last life, we were married and lived happily ever after until I went and got myself shot. Yeah, that's just not gonna fly.

He spent the next few days trying to find a casual way to run into her, with no success. He came to know her neighborhood as well as his own back in Emeryville.

So, what am I now, Emily's stalker? I guess so, but this is different. We love each other, or at least we have loved each other, and I believe we will again. Unless, of course, this is all part of some delusion I've been living in since I got shot. Maybe I'm really lying in a coma at a hospital in Middle Falls in 1999.

Dominick learned what Emily's schedule was over the next week—what time she went to class, and what time she got out. After that, he gave up staking out her house, but he still tried to position himself to run into her on campus.

On the Friday of his first week in town, he walked into the Student Union Building again, trying to reconnoiter the layout. Just as he reached the door, Emily pushed it open, heading out. He swung the door wide and tried to come up with something, anything to say, but he was completely tongue-tied. She pushed past him, smiled casually, and said, "Thank you."

"Don't mention it," was all that came out.

Emily got to her car and drove away.

Don't mention it. Don't mention it?! Moron! Why not, "Happy to open the door for a beautiful woman?" Probably because that would make me sound like a low-rent Pepe Le Pew.

That night, Dominick laid on top of the twin bed in his makeshift room, thinking.

I really believed this would be easy—that if I was ever in her presence, that somehow, some vestige of "us" would be there, that she would recognize me on some level. Instead, she walks right by me like I am a complete stranger. Which, I guess I am.

Dominick rolled over on the thin, uncomfortable mattress, trying to find a comfortable way to lay on it.

I could try and prove to her that I already know her. Tell her that I know her guilty pleasure is listening to Barry Manilow records, or that she loves to hoard and eat Pixie Stix in bed, or that she cries every time she watches It's a Wonderful Life? *Nah. Everyone loves Manilow, Pixie Stix, and Jimmy Stewart movies, right? If I told her I knew about that cute little birthmark on her inner thigh it probably wouldn't go over well, either. I'd probably end up meeting that cop again.*

Another week passed. That Friday afternoon, Dominick sat slumped behind the wheel of his car, half-heartedly reading a used copy of *The Grapes of Wrath* he had picked up at the book store downtown. Over the top of the book, movement caught his eye and he saw it was Emily and the two girls she was so often with, emerging from the Student Union. Dominick had dubbed the other two girls Debbie One and Debbie Two. Debbie One was a shorter brunette, cute and curvy. Debbie Two was another blonde, like Emily, but not nearly as pretty, especially in Dominick's eyes.

They got into the same station wagon that Emily always drove, and headed away from campus. Dominick followed along, berating himself for being such a stalker, but unable to help himself.

I can't do this much longer. I'll go crazy.

Dominick didn't even bother to follow the station wagon. He could tell by the route, they were doing what they always did—heading for Emily's house. Dominick took a side trip to The Point Drive In for a burger and frozen custard, a new habit he had picked up.

After that, he gassed up the Chevy and thought of heading back to what passed for home at the moment. The thought of the blanket-walled room was too depressing to think about, so he followed the path he had taken so often – back to Emily's house.

Just as he passed her house, he saw a car he'd never seen there before—a late sixties Mustang—pull out of the driveway. He could see at least four people inside, and figured that Emily was likely among them.

Maybe they'll end up at a place where I can find a way to have an actual conversation with her.

The Mustang was in no hurry, and was easy to follow as it wound through neighborhoods sticking to surface streets and avoiding the freeway. Eventually it pulled into a parking lot with a sign out front that read, "Sheboygan Falls Lanes." A neon bowling ball rolled into three neon pins, over and over.

Dominick turned into the parking lot behind them, but parked in a far off corner. By the time he shut off the car and walked toward where the Mustang was, it was empty. He walked through the double doors that led into the bowling alley. The smell of the aerosol sprayed into hundreds of pairs of bowling shoes, the wax on the lanes, and hot grease from the food court combined into the unmistakable *eau du bowling alley* smell that was familiar to just about everyone. A cloud of bluish smoke from a thousand cigarettes hung over the entire place.

Dominick looked around and spotted Debbie One and Debbie Two putting on their bowling shoes at lane sixteen. Emily was nowhere in sight. He walked to the bowling counter, which came more than halfway up his chest.

Why the heck do they always make these counters so high? To give someone handing out shoes a sense of power?

Dominick asked for a pair of size ten and a half shoes.

The man behind the counter stubbed out a cigarette in an ashtray overflowing with the burned bodies of its comrades. He blew a cloud of smoke toward Dominick and said, "How many games?"

"How much per game?"

"Forty cents a line, or three for a dollar. Fifty cents for the shoes."

"I'll take three games," Dominick said, and laid a dollar bill and two quarters down on the counter. He smoothed an extra dollar out on the counter. "Can you give me lane fifteen?

The counterman looked at the dollar, glanced out at lane sixteen, where Debbie Two was rolling a gutter ball. The extra dollar disappeared. "I'll put you on lane fifteen, then."

Dominick picked up the red and tan shoes and walked to the ball rack, looking for a ball with the proper finger grip. As he did, he saw Emily come from the direction of the snack bar. She was walking next to a guy with blond hair, a wispy mustache, and a big smile on his face. They were holding hands.

Chapter Thirty-Three

Dominick stumbled to one of the plastic chairs that was sitting next to the ball rack. Emily and the man Dominick suddenly wanted to kill walked by him without so much as a glance. They joined the other two girls and sat around the lane, talking, not seeming too worried about bowling.

Dominick's heart was thudding in his chest. His palms were sweating, and his knees were weak.

Of course. Of course she has a boyfriend. How could she not? She's so smart, so pretty, so Emily, *of course everyone here would fall in love with her just like I did.* Dominick took a deep breath and held it before letting it hiss out between his teeth. *Certainly complicates things, though.*

Dominick watched the foursome, heads together, telling some private joke, then leaning back, laughing and laughing.

I think I might throw up.

Dominick stood up, steadied himself, and returned to the search for a ball that fit his hand. After a few tries, he found a psychedelic green and orange splattered ball that worked.

Now I wish I hadn't tipped the guy to get right next to them.

Dominick stepped onto lane fifteen and sat the ball down in the proper spot, then sat at the left-hand scoring table. Debbie Two had turned around and was writing their names on the scoresheet.

Dominick glanced over and saw that she had written, "Melody," "Sandy," "Emily," and "Burke," down the left hand side of the sheet.

Burke. Burke? What the hell kind of name is Burke? That sounds like the name of a kid that got beat up a lot in grade school.

The girl, whose name was apparently either Melody or Sandy, glanced over at Dominick. "If you're gonna peep on us, the least you can do is write your name down, so we know who's stalking us."

Dominick let out a nervous laugh. "Oh, ha, ha, stalking, ha, ha." He realized that he might be sounding a little crazy, and that she was likely just joking. "Sorry. I'm Dominick."

"Hi. I'm Sandy. This is Melody over here, and the two lovebirds behind us are Burke and Emily."

Dominick glanced over his shoulder. Both Burke and Emily smiled at him. Melody said, "Well, hello, foxy. What's a nice boy like you doing in a bowling alley like this?"

Dominick blushed a little, shrugged, and searched for a smile he couldn't find. He stood up to bowl. He was a good athlete, good at almost every sport he ever tried. Except bowling. Somehow his body just didn't get the hang of the approach, the release, the spin of the ball. He walked to the first set of arrows, lined up just to the right of the pocket, and did his best to send a ball whizzing triumphantly into the pins. Instead, it hooked badly, and just managed to nick the 7 pin on the way by.

Dominick rolled his shoulders, cricked his neck, and put his fingers over the hand dryer, waiting for the ball to return. When it finally clunked out of the ball return, he went through the same routine. Unremarkably, that produced the same result, except this time there was no 7 pin to knock down.

Chagrined, Dominick returned to the scorecard, and without sitting down, marked a "1" in the first frame.

"You have come to the right place, boychik. None of us are auditioning for the Pro Bowler's Tour, either," Sandy said.

"Thanks."

After a few frames, Dominick went to the snack bar for a soda and a bag of chips. When he returned, he sat and watched the foursome bowl. Sandy was right—none of them were much better as bowlers. But being so near Emily, watching her graceful movements as she bowled, then smelling her perfume as she walked past him on her way to sit next to *Burke*, to hold his hand, to whisper in his ear, was torture.

Beyond that first smile, neither Emily nor Burke seemed to even notice Dominick. Melody, on the other hand, was more than a little interested. When Dominick sat down to record a score, she would often lean over to say something to him, pushing her shoulder into his. She was very cute, with dark, bouncy hair done in a Dorothy Hamill flip, flashing dark brown eyes, and an ever-present grin. In another life, a life before he had met Emily, Dominick would have been flattered by her attention.

Here, in this situation, where all he wanted to do was strangle Burke and sit down for a forty year conversation with Emily, it only meant trouble.

You'd think that living a life for a second time would make everything easier. So, why does it seem to get more complicated instead?

Dominick finished his second game while the four of them finished their first. He decided to forfeit the third game and get out of there. He had accomplished one goal—to get close to Emily in a social situation, and absolutely nothing had come of it. In fact, he was much further behind the eight ball than he had been. Emily had a boyfriend and, no matter how hard he tried—and he had listened like a hawk listening for a mouse's rustling—he couldn't hear Burke say anything lousy. In fact, he seemed like a pretty decent guy, aside from the fact that he was holding Emily's hand, and occasionally kissing her. On top of that, one of her friends—Melody, as it turned out, not Debbie One—seemed to like him.

So, how can I tell Melody, "You're a great girl, but I really want to get with your friend, who, by the way, already has a boyfriend."

He sat in the molded plastic chair, took his bowling shoes off and put his Chuck Taylors back on. He grabbed his scoresheet, on which he had recorded scores of 92 and 112, and prepared to toss it away. As he did, Melody leaned over and said, "Hey, not to be too forward or anything, but what are you doing later on tonight?"

Her breath smells like cherry-flavored bubble gum.

Dominick was caught completely off guard, and stuttered for a moment before saying, "Ummm ...nothing."

"We're going to go to a midnight screening of a movie called *Rocky Horror Picture Show*. It's kind of a blast. Do you want to come with us?"

Wow, she said that like Rocky *is new, which I guess it probably is, in 1977 Sheboygan.*

Dominick looked at Melody, her big brown eyes questioning him. He could see that asking him to go with her had cost her something.

"Sure. Where?"

"It's playing at the Lakeside."

"Okay, sure."

"We get there a little early – around eleven. Burke does this weird thing where local people get up and mime along with the movie."

Of course he does. Dominick looked at Burke with new eyes. Tall, strongly built, blond hair, shorter on top, but curling over the collar of his shirt in back. *Were they shadow casting in the upper Midwest in 1977? I guess so, here's the evidence.*

"We meet at a little café called *BJ's*, just down the street, for coffee. You want to meet us there?"

Dominick smiled, a slightly sick little smile, and nodded. "I'll be there."

He returned his ball to the rack, picked up his bowling shoes, grabbed his jacket and headed for the counter. On the way by Emily and Burke, he nodded. They both gave him a little wave, but didn't notice it made his lip curl back away from his teeth.

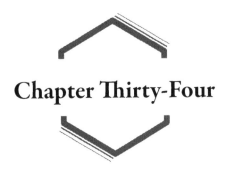

Chapter Thirty-Four

Dominick drove home and tucked himself away in his little basement hideaway. He pulled all his clothes out of his duffel bag, wondering if he should change, but decided to go with the Levi's and baby blue *Keep on Truckin'* t-shirt he had worn bowling.

He sat on the edge of his bed and tried to figure out where he had gone wrong. By the time he left, he had a two part plan: first, separate himself from Melody and next, separate Emily from Burke. The first was probably easy, but he had no idea how to accomplish the second.

He had driven by the Lakeside Theater a number of times, so he knew how to get there. It was a cold, rainy, late September night, with puddles littering the streets. The inside of the Chevelle's windows kept fogging up. Soon enough, though, he saw the lighted marquee of the Lakeside. According to the marquee, *Star Wars* had played at 8:00. In smaller letters at the bottom, it said, *Rocky Horror Midnight*. A block beyond the theater, he spotted the warm light of BJ's Diner and pulled into their little parking lot. Through the front window, Dominick could see the four of them, sitting around a table, drinking coffee.

If I just turn around and drive away they couldn't find me. He turned off his headlights and windshield wipers, but left the car running. *And then what would I do? How could I ever talk to Emily? At least this way, I'll be close to Emily, being eaten alive by jealousy.*

Dominick turned the ignition off, flipped up the collar of his bomber jacket and headed inside. The diner was so brightly lit, it made him squint when he opened the door. Both Melody and Sandy spotted him and waved him over. They pulled out a chair right between them.

Dominick sat down and immediately became the focus of everyone at the table, including Emily. She led off the questioning.

"So, Mr. Dominick, just exactly what are your intentions regarding our Miss Melody, here?"

Dominick tried to find his smart ass attitude that was so often on display, but failed. "Umm, just here to catch the movie, I think."

Emily laughed, and put her hand over his for a moment. Her touch was electric and warmed him all the way through. He glanced at her eyes to see if she felt it, too, but if she did, she showed no sign. "Just kidding around. She's a grown up lady. She can do whoever, I mean, whatever, she wants." She finished with a wink at Melody, who didn't seem embarrassed in the slightest.

Across the table, Burke shrugged, a silent acknowledgment that he is definitely not in charge. "Do you go to UW?" he asked.

Dominick shook his head. "No, I'm from out of state."

Emily's eyes lit up. "Oh, a visitor to our fair land. Where are you from?"

"California," Dominick said, and all the girls sighed together.

"Hollywood?" Melody asked.

"No, but that would be a much cooler answer. I grew up in Emeryville, in northern California, not too far from San Francisco."

Burke leaned forward a bit. "What in the world would pull you away from the West Coast and drop you in Wisconsin? Gotta be a girl, right?"

Dominick's eyes shifted involuntarily toward Emily, but he quickly looked away. He smiled, and said, "No, I just graduated from high school, and I want to see the country before I buckle down and start college."

"So," Burke said, "our whole wide nation spreads out before you, and you end up in the Bratwurst Capital of the World? I think your compass is broken."

Dominick laughed it off. "I just want to take a couple of years and travel everywhere, see a little bit of everything." *This isn't going all that well.* "So, I've never heard of this movie we're going to see. What's it about?"

"Oh, it's a blast," Melody said, pressing against Dominick. "It's freaky and fun, and the audience is part of the show, too. Burke is part of it. He plays Rocky."

Of course he does. I just can't wait to see him in the gold bikini brief. Blech.

Melody produced a grocery bag from underneath the table. "We've got everything we need for the show—squirt guns, toast, and newspapers. Don't worry, I'll be right beside you. I'll show you everything you need to do."

Burke, in a conspiratorial faux-whisper, said, "Not the first time she's said that to a guy."

"Hush, Burke," Emily said, but she was smiling, too.

Burke stood up. "Well, there's a cast meeting that's starting right now, so I've gotta run. See you guys over there." He bent down and kissed Emily for several long seconds as Dominick felt his stomach tie in knots.

"So," Dominick said, just to have something to say, "Are all you guys students at UW? What are you studying?"

"Yeah, but we're mostly just getting our prerequisites out of the way. Our parents aren't rich, and it costs a lot more to go to Madison, because of the cost of housing," Emily said, "My parents are cool. They told me they'd cover my tuition either way, but if I went to Madison, I'd have to get a job to pay for a dorm or off-campus apartment. I decided to do both. So, I've got a job that starts in a few weeks, and I'm going to stay home and save for the first two years, then finish up in Madison."

Typical Emily. Give her two choices, she'll always find the third, and it's always better. Typical of Harvey and Louise, too. Kind, but firm. And smart. They were the best in-laws I could have asked for.

Dominick turned to Sandy and Melody. "How about you guys?"

Melody pointed at Sandy. "She's just trolling for a well-off husband, I think. And me? I have no idea what I am going to do."

The four of them chatted comfortably for a few more minutes, then left a couple of dollars on the table for the coffees and made their way to the theater.

Dominick had seen *Rocky Horror* a number of times, but not for close to twenty years, when he had seen the Portland Shadow cast at the Clinton Street Theater. The cast here in Sheboygan wasn't as good, but it was all new to them, and they gave it their all, no matter how many missed cues or flubbed lines they had. As usual, the crowd, and the insults it flung at the screen, were the best part of the show.

By the time the Lakeside Theater manager had made his preshow announcement, complete with catcalls of "Boring!," the music video of *Love Stinks* by The J. Geils Band, and the movie itself, it was after 2:00 am before the house lights came up. Throughout the movie, Melody had been a constant presence next to Dominick, sitting close to him, leaning over to show him what to do, trying to teach him the callbacks. Dominick did everything he could to extricate himself without being too obvious about it. By the end of the movie, she wasn't trying as hard.

When the movie was over, and the crowd was spilling out into the cold Wisconsin night, Melody grabbed Dominick and said, "I drove myself tonight, so my car is back at the diner. Walk me there?"

Dominick nodded and said, "Of course."

As they walked, Melody reached out and put her arm through Dominick's. When they got to her car, she turned to him, "We're not gonna happen, are we?"

She's a great girl, and so sweet. She deserves to know.

Dominick smiled back sadly and shook his head.

"Thanks for letting me know. That's better. Any particular reason? Did I forget to brush my teeth this morning?"

Dominick laughed a little. "You're so cool, Melody. You're a beautiful girl, and I know you could get just about any guy you want."

"Unless that guy is you..." her words, and her thought, trailed off into nothingness.

"There's another girl that I really care about, but I can't be with her right now. It just wouldn't feel right."

There. That's about as close to the truth as I can get.

She looked at him appraisingly, letting possibilities tumble over and over in her mind. Finally, she said, "That's what I need, what I'd love to find—someone who feels like that about me. Thanks for being honest."

"I hope you guys will still let me hang out with you, I think you're all great, and I don't know anyone else in the entire state."

"Of course we will. But, one word of advice. If you're gonna keep stalking someone, you shouldn't drive a cherry-red Super Sport. It kind of stands out and we've been watching you for a week now. I just figured it was me you were after. No such luck."

Dominick's mouth fell open. Melody stood on her tiptoes and kissed his cheek, hurried into her car and left.

I am never even half as smart as I think I am.

Chapter Thirty-Five

Carrie expertly finessed her pyxis, jumping from one life she oversaw to another. She felt an obligation to all the people she watched over, but she found herself spending more time on those she felt the strongest connection with.

She tuned in to Michael Hollister, sitting on a couch in his quiet quarters, reading a book, with a short, round-faced man sitting beside him watching television.

This life was so hectic for him, but now it's settled down into a steady routine, marked off with military precision. She moved the focus onto his face. The only movement was Michael's eyes across the page of the book and the flames of the fire in the fireplace. *Good for you, Michael. You deserve it.*

She moved the pyxis again, catching glimpses of different lives, at different places on their own time continuum, but nothing caught her interest. She let the image come to rest on a picture of five young people sitting around a table in a café, drinking coffee. They were laughing and talking, but there was nothing unusual or interesting about the scene. Two of them—the dark-haired boy and the pretty blonde girl with the heart-shaped face—were both hers.

They've been together before, they'll be together again. I just can't tell if it's for good or not.

Carrie reached out to move on again, when she heard Bertellia's voice say, "Oh, Emillion. How nice to see her."

Carrie was startled. Her supervisor so rarely initiated a conversation with her, and when she did, it was usually to grill her over something. "I'm sorry?"

"Oh, the blonde girl there. That's Emillion. I've known her for millennia."

Carrie pointed to the girl. "Her? That's Emily."

"Yes," Bertellia said, then moved on between the rows of desks.

Chapter Thirty-Six

For the next three months, Dominick continued to hang out regularly with Emily, Burke, Melody, and Sandy. They called themselves *The Fearsome Fivesome*, and life went on. Dominick got a job as a pump jockey for a Texaco station. It paid just a bit over minimum wage—$2.95 an hour—but he had done the math, and even living frugally, he knew he would soon run out of money if he didn't have an income of some sort.

Emily and Burke continued to live a momentary happily-ever-after, at least to Dominick's eyes. As much as he hated it, he had to admit that Burke was a good guy. He and Dominick even hung out on their own a few times, playing a game of pickup hoops at UW, or catching an action movie that none of the girls wanted to see.

Dominick continued to live in his blanket fort in Gene Crow's basement. Crow had promised to put real walls up, but months after Dominick had moved in, there had been no movement on that front. Dominick knew that if Crow ever did put the walls up, his rent would almost double, so kept his mouth shut about it.

Dominick called home every week, just as he had promised. Connie was always glad to talk to him, full of stories of high school dances and cute new boys, but both Joe and Laura were confused and more than a little frustrated by his continued stay in Wisconsin.

A pre-Christmas phone call home was typical.

"We just don't understand, Nicky. It's Christmas time. You should be home with us," Louise said.

"I know, Mom. I'll be back eventually."

Joe took the phone. "I could understand it if you were going to school, or in a career, or even if you were just being a beach bum in Florida. But you're pumping gas and washing windshields in Wisconsin, for God's sake. Help us understand."

But of course, Dominick couldn't help them understand. He couldn't say, "I'm here watching what I hope is my future wife canoodle with her boyfriend, and hanging out with two other cute girls I have absolutely no interest in."

Snowfall was common in Sheboygan in December, but in 1977, a major storm hit that nearly closed the city down for four days. A rear wheel drive Chevelle, nimble under normal conditions, became a severe liability on frozen and snow covered streets, so Dominick relied on Sheboygan Transit, such as it was, when he was forced to leave the house to work.

In the midst of the storm, Melody called him at the boarding house. Dominick had been afraid she might act cool or distant to him after their date at *Rocky Horror*, but she hadn't been. If anything, she teased him more brutally after that—about being a snobby Californian, a bookworm, a loser with no love life, whatever came to her mind.

Dominick was laying on his bed, reading a Ray Bradbury novel, when Gene Crow's booming voice came down the stairwell. "Davidner! Phone!"

Dominick tensed, knowing what was next. Sure enough, as he made his way to the top of the stairs, Crow was there, holding the door open. "The house phone is really for emergencies. We can't tie it up for personal chit chat." He said exactly the same thing, every time anyone got a call, even if it was the first call they had received after living there for months.

Dominick nodded and waved at him on the way to the phone, which sat on a towering pile of fashion magazines and junk mail. "Hello?"

"Hey, Nicky," Melody said. She had asked Dominick what his family called him, and his name had changed, at least to her, immediately.

"Hey, Mel. How's the outside world?"

"Snowy."

"What a coinkeedink. Same here."

"Wanna come over to Emily's place?"

"I don't think my car will make it. It's buried in a drift three feet high."

"I've got my dad's four wheel drive. I'll come pick you up. Everybody's scattering for Christmas soon, so this is our last chance to all get together for a while."

Dominick had small presents for everyone already wrapped, so he said, "Okay, that works. You know where I live?"

"Of course I do. You're not the only stalker, stalker. See you at 4:00, okay?"

"Sure. Come around to the side door, though, okay? It's a long story." Dominick said goodbye, then hung up and went back downstairs to wait.

Melody wasn't an on-time kind of girl. She was more the type to keep boys waiting, even if they weren't dating. She arrived for her 4:00 pickup at 4:38 sharp. When she knocked on the side door, two of the other tenants were in the kitchen, warming up a frozen pizza, and making Ramen noodles, respectively.

Melody bustled in, wearing a miniskirt and a smile that lit up even that depressing room, and asked for Dominick. Based on their reactions to Melody, his stock obviously had gone up several notches in the eyes of his roommates. One of them, a UW student named

Mark, shouted down the stairs, "Dude, there's a girl here asking for you, and she's cuter than hell."

Dominick grabbed his coat, small armful of gifts, and bounced up the stairs to rescue her from the stares of his roomies. They climbed into her Dad's Bronco and pulled out into the non-existent traffic.

Melody drove as she did so many other things in life—without a care in the world. That was fine, in perfect weather. In near-blizzard conditions, being in the passenger seat became an exercise in courage. She bounced along from one rut to another, sliding a bit here, fishtailing a bit there, singing along with Brenda Lee and *Rockin' Around the Christmas Tree* the entire time.

"Ummm, Mel?"

"Yeah?"

"You know that four wheel drive doesn't actually make you invincible, right? Sometimes, it just means that you've got four tires spinning instead of two."

Melody laughed, switched the radio station, and tapped the steering wheel in time with the new song. "You worry too much."

"I think maybe you don't worry enough! Like, where the nearest hospital is, if you severely injure your innocent passenger."

After a white knuckle ride, they arrived at Emily's with everything intact except Dominick's nerves. Walking up the front steps of Emily's house, Dominick's stomach flipped. He was almost used to seeing Emily by now, but he hadn't met her parents in this life. The last time he had seen them, they had been two retirees traveling the country in their RV and making a side trip to Middle Falls, Oregon.

Melody didn't ring the bell, but threw the door open and bounced into the hallway, saying, "Mom, Dad, I'm home!"

A woman who appeared to be in her early fifties came around the corner, wiping her hands on a dishrag. She had blonde hair streaked through with gray. Something about her made Dominick like her immediately. Again.

Hello, Louise.

"Hello, Melody, who's this you've brought with you?"

Dominick stepped forward and said, "Hi, I'm Dominick. I'm a friend of Mel and Emily."

"Oh, you're Dominick. How nice. I've been hearing a lot about you. Louise Esterhaus. Very nice to meet you."

"Emily in her room?" Melody asked.

Louise nodded. "Go on back. She's there with Burke and Sandy."

Burke. Yippee.

They went down the hall to a bedroom on the left. They went in and Dominick stopped dead. Emily, Burke, and Sandy were all lounging around the room. A small record player in the corner was playing a 45 of the Eagles *Please Come Home for Christmas*. One entire wall was covered in paintings and drawings. He gawked at them.

Everyone looked at him and laughed. "Yeah," Emily said, "It's a little crazy, I know."

Every painting was different, but there was something that connected all of them. They looked like images that might be used on the cover of a science fiction novel. One painting was a large landscape with alien trees bending over an inky ocean, three moons hanging in the sky above. Another showed a massive city with architecture that had never been seen on Earth, with swooping lines and towering spires. Among the paintings were charcoal drawings that looked like concept drawings for other fantastical realms.

"What ... who did all these?"

"I did," Emily said, with a mixture of shyness and pride.

Emily, I always knew you liked to dabble, but I never knew you could do this. Why did I not know?

"They're amazing. Mind blowing." Dominick stepped up to one for a closer look. "The detail is incredible. Did you ... copy them from somewhere?"

As soon as he said it, he thought Emily might take offense, but she didn't. She just shook her head. "I don't know where all this stuff comes from. Sometimes I dream about places. Other times, I guess I just feel like I'm there. I don't feel like I am making things up, I'm just painting what I see."

"Amazing. Are you studying art?"

"No, Mom and Dad would never go for that. I'm either going to major in Accounting, or go for my teaching degree. Haven't decided yet."

"Hey, guys," Sandy said. "Everyone sit on the bed for me, K?"

Emily and Burke scooted over and made room for Dominick and Melody.

Sandy pulled a Polaroid camera out of a bag. She pushed a flash bar into place. "Now, say 'cheese!'"

No one said cheese. Instead, everyone stuck their tongue out at her. She pushed a button, the flash went off, and acrid smoke puffed up. A whirr followed, as a picture ejected itself from the camera.

"Now, one where everyone doesn't look cross-eyed, please."

The four of them gave a relatively normal smile, and the camera produced another flash of light and smoke.

Melody started to get up, but Dominick said, "Hey, would you take one that I could have?"

"Yeah, of course! Positions!"

Another flash, another puff, and a third picture ejected from the camera. Sandy took it, shook it, and handed it to Dominick. "Merry Christmas."

The best Christmas present I can imagine is a picture of Emily. Now, I just have to wait another decade or two for Photoshop to be invented, so I can erase Burke out of the picture.

Melody elbowed Dominick. "Speaking of Merry Christmas, are you the kind of guy who brings a bunch of presents with you, then doesn't give them out, or what?"

Dominick looked at the small pile of presents. "Oh, right. I forgot. It's not much. I just wanted to get you guys something. I don't know what I would have done without you the last couple of months. Probably would have gone crazy."

He handed a present to everyone. Typical teenagers, no one was embarrassed that they didn't have anything for him. Dominick had done all his shopping in one place, *One More Chapter*, the used bookstore down by the college.

"I know not everyone is a reader, but I tried to find something you might like."

Or, to be honest, I found three books for three of you, so I could give one book to Emily without raising eyebrows.

"One at a time, please," Emily said. "I love to watch people open presents."

Sandy opened a copy of *Giants in the Earth*, by Hans Rolvaag. "I got that for you, because you said you love the *Little House on the Prairie* books. This is like that, only even better."

"Thank you, but of course, nothing can be better than *Little House*. Still, I love it. Thank you." She leaned over and hugged Dominick.

Burke opened a copy of the previous year's *Guinness Book of World Records*. "I figured that would help you win a few bar bets, if you memorized it."

Burke waved the book at him, and said, "Thank you, man. Very cool."

Melody tore the wrapping off hers, to reveal a copy of Robert Heinlein's *Stranger in a Strange Land*. She looked quizzically at it, then opened the cover to read the inscription: *To Melody, my Water Brother, from Dominick, Christmas, 1977.*

"I don't know how to tell you this, Mr. Davidner," she said, thrusting her shoulders back and pushing her chest forward, "but I am no one's brother."

Dominick laughed, and said, "Once you read the book you'll understand. It's a term of endearment, and friendship, and trust."

"I trust you," she said seriously and planted a kiss on his cheek that tingled with warmth.

Dominick took a deep breath, turned to Emily, and said, "Your turn."

"I can't wait to see what you think I would read," she said, sliding her finger along the tape and slipping a thin book out of the wrapping.

I cheated, Em. I bought you your all-time favorite book, you just don't know it yet, because it just came out, and you wouldn't have found it for another year. I'm willing to cheat a little when it comes to you.

Emily turned the book over. *Illusions, The Adventures of a Reluctant Messiah* by Richard Bach.

A question crossed her face.

"I know you've never heard of it. It just came out, but I read it, and it just made me think of you."

If Burke was bothered by this familiarity with his girlfriend, he didn't show it.

She opened it. On the first page, Dominick had written, "*Your friends will know you better in the first minute, than your acquaintances will know you in a thousand years.*"

"Did you write that?" Now Burke leaned his head over, so he could see the inscription.

"No. I'm not that smart. It's from the book."

"What's it about?"

"Well, it's about a man who flies around the country, giving people rides in his old bi-wing airplane. He meets a man who may or may not be a modern day messiah. You'll have to read it and decide on whether he is or not for yourself."

And I already know the answer, as you had a small, blue feather tattooed on your hip. Very un-school marm-ish, Teach. I love you, Emily, and I'm so glad I get to give you that book. I hope you will think about this moment and smile, every time you read it.

Three days later, back at BJ's, with cups of hot chocolate steaming in front of them, Emily leaned across the table to Dominick. "*Illusions* was the most amazing book I've ever read. I don't know what made you think to give it to me, but thank you. I've read it twice already, and I bet I'll read a hundred more times in my lifetime."

Dominick nearly pulled a Han Solo, and said, "I know," but he checked himself. He looked into her never to be forgotten gray eyes, and said, "Good. I got lucky."

Chapter Thirty-Seven

Three months later, life was still unchanged for Dominick. He worked at the gas station five days a week. He made enough there that he wasn't depleting his savings any more, but he wasn't getting ahead, either. He was also bored stiff, doing the same menial tasks over and over again.

He was beyond frustrated with his relationship, or lack thereof, with Emily. The Fearsome Fivesome hung out as much as ever, sometimes going places, most often just sitting together in someone's bedroom, listening to music and talking. Dominick liked all of them—even Burke—but being so close to Emily, yet so far from the relationship he wanted to have with her, was driving him to distraction.

They even came to Dominick's place. The first time they did, Melody led them to the side door. Dominick had never seen the front door of the house actually open, although beyond Crow's Obsessive Compulsive Disorder, he didn't know the reason for it. Unfortunately, it was Gene Crow who answered the side door the day everyone showed up. He made Emily, Melody, and Sandy so uncomfortable that Burke had stepped in front of them.

"Can you just show us where Dominick is, please?"

Crow waved a hand in the general direction of the stairs, but didn't take his eyes off the girls. When they found Dominick's makeshift room, the first thing Sandy said was, "Oh my God, you live in a blanket fort!" Then, she added, "And I don't ever want that man to look at me again. His eyes were handsier than a senior on prom night. He was undressing me from across the room." Sandy and Emily agreed.

Inside his room, they noticed the window above his bed.

"Does that open?" Burke asked.

"Yeah, it slides open. Why?"

"Because next time we hang out here, we should just all come around and drop down onto your bed."

"Great idea," Melody said. "But I won't wear a short skirt when I do."

EVERYTHING CHANGED one Tuesday afternoon in March. Melody had stopped by the service station just as his shift ended. "What time do you get off?"

Dominick eyed the *Put a Tiger in your tank* wall clock, and said, "Not long. Maybe twenty minutes."

"I'll wait."

"What's up?"

"Emily and Burke broke up."

The blood drained from Dominick's face. He did his best to keep his voice steady. "What?"

"Yeah, Emily just broke up with Burke. She called and told me. She sounds okay, but I think she might need us around. So, get going gas jockey!"

Dominick wiped his hands on a rag, went to the office and told his boss, Sal, that he needed to knock off a few minutes early—that he had a small emergency.

Sal looked out his office door at Melody, dressed that day in a pair of tight jeans and a warm sweater, and said, "That's the kind of small emergency we all need in our lives. Get it while you're young."

Dominick opened his mouth to explain, but instead said, "Great, Sal. Thanks. I'll be here first thing tomorrow for my shift."

"With a smile on your face, no doubt."

Dominick jumped in the Chevelle and headed to Emily's with Melody in the lead. When they pulled in front of the house, Dominick noticed that Sandy's car was already there, but Burke's Mustang was nowhere in sight.

Dominick got to the front door first, but waited for Melody. Even after a dozen visits, he wasn't prepared to just blow in with a jaunty, "Hi, Mom!" like Melody did.

They let themselves in and made their way back to Emily's room. They found Em and Sandy, sitting on the bed, leaning back against the wall. The anthem for every seventies breakup, Carol King's *Tapestry*, was playing on the stereo.

Dominick's heart leapt at the sight of Emily. *There's no reason in the world we can't be together, now. Can you see me now, like I see you?*

Dominick sat crossed-legged on the floor, and Melody scrunched down into the orange bean bag chair beside him.

"So, what's up, chickie?"

Emily shrugged, and Dominick saw that although she was clear-eyed, there was sadness there.

Take it easy, take it easy.

Finally, after everyone had finished listening to Carol King sing *So Far Away*, Emily said, "Burke just has his whole life planned out. He's known since fourth grade that he was going to go to college and study architecture, just like his dad. He knew from our second date that we were going to get married. He knew exactly when we were going to start having kids. He even knew what we were going to name them."

That was an arrow through Dominick's heart. *We tried, but we were never able to.*

"That's all great, but I'm eighteen years old. I have no idea what I want to do with my life. The only thing I'm sure of right now is that I don't want to make up my mind today. I just want to live first."

Sandy leaned her head over against Emily's shoulder and took her hand.

"The thing is," Emily continued, "I can't help but wonder. Am I blowing it? Burke's a really good guy. He's smart, and kind, and I love his parents, and ... I don't know. Should I hold it against him that he has his shit together?"

Dominick hadn't said a word. He felt a little out of place there, as if his maleness was intruding on the sanctity of a female bonding experience. He cleared his throat.

"You want to know what I think?"

Emily looked at him as if she was realizing he was there for the first time. She nodded.

"I think you need to listen to the small voice you hear inside yourself when no one else is around. That's your intuition, telling you what to do." *As long as it's not telling you that you made a mistake and to go running back to Burke.*

"You're so wise, California-boy," Melody said, patting his knee.

"No, it's just my answer to everything. It's how I ended up here, in this room, with you guys."

DOMINICK KNEW THAT the first few weeks after Emily's breakup were critical.

Don't want to jump in too soon, like a shark circling for blood in the water. But, I also don't want to meet everybody one night and find Emily holding hands with some dude who didn't know she had just broken up with her boyfriend and asked her out.

Dominick just enjoyed being the only man in the trusted inner circle of Emily, Melody and Sandy for a month.

Finally, he couldn't take it anymore. The thought of Emily, just a few miles away, likely doing nothing in particular, was too much for him. He went upstairs to the main floor at Crow Mansion, looked around to see if Gene Crow was nearby—he didn't want another lecture about the phone again—then went into the dining room, picked up the heavy black receiver and dialed Emily's number from memory.

After a few rings, Louise Esterhaus answered. "Hello?"

"Greetings, Mrs. Esterhaus."

"Louise," she corrected. "Hello, Dominick."

"Sorry. Louise. Is Emily there?"

"Sure. Hang on."

Dominick heard the phone clump down on the counter and Louise calling Emily. A click as Emily picked up the pink princess phone in her room, then another as Louise hung up the kitchen phone. She was not the type to spy on her daughter's calls.

"Hello?"

"Hey, Em. It's Dominick." *It's such a miracle to be able to say those words.*

His hands went suddenly slick, and his breath seemed to catch in his throat. *This is ridiculous. We were married for ten years. I know everything about you. There's nothing to be nervous about.*

He wiped his hands against his jeans.

"Hey, what's up?"

What's up is, I love you. I have loved you from the first moment I saw you in my first lifetime. Now, we've been apart for ten years. You don't know it, but I do, and I feel the weight of our absence. I want to spend every day of the rest of our lives with you.

"Not much. Just wondering if you wanted to hang out tonight?"

"Umm, sure. You want me to call Mel and Sandy?"

"No, not really."

Silence hung in the air for two beats, then three. "Oh." That single syllable came out as soft as a feather pillow. It spoke of a realization that the direction of the wind had changed.

Dominick started to lose his nerve. "Would that be okay? If it's not, I understand."

Hollow silence, broken by small bursts of static stretched into what felt like an eternity to Dominick.

Finally, strong and clear, Emily said, "No, that would be good. Nice."

What we had wasn't just nice, *Emily. It changed my whole life. But, for now, I will take it.*

"How about if I pick you up in an hour? Maybe we can just go to BJ's and have some coffee and split an order of their fries?"

"Sounds good. See you then."

Dominick slipped the phone back into the cradle.

DOMINICK PULLED INTO Emily's driveway less than an hour later, but she must have been watching for him, because she came out before he even had a chance to turn the Chevelle off.

She slid into the passenger seat and said, "Nice wheels, Nicky."

He feigned surprise. "What, have you never been in my car before?" *I know you haven't. You always rode with Burke or Mel.*

He drove slowly to BJ's. It was raining steadily, but the windshield wipers slapping back and forth just added to the coziness of being alone with Emily. When he turned into the parking lot, the steady rain turned into a downpour.

"Let's wait it out," Dominick said.

"If you don't like Wisconsin weather in the springtime, just wait five minutes. It'll change."

Small talk.

Dominick turned around in his seat. The rain thrummed a rhythm against the roof. It was cold outside, but very warm inside.

Emily turned slightly and stared at him, wide-eyed.

Calm washed over Dominick.

Ever so slowly, giving Emily a thousand chances to pull away, he leaned toward her.

She did not pull away, but leaned toward him slightly.

He closed his eyes, and when his lips met hers, he knew he was exactly where he belonged.

Chapter Thirty-Eight

The next few months were among the happiest of Dominick's two lives. The only dark cloud on his horizon was trying to explain to his parents why he had set off from California to see the world, and, nine months later, had made it to Sheboygan, Wisconsin and no further.

Finally, a month after he and Emily had officially been an item—their official coming out occurring when they revealed their 'couplehood' to Melody and Sandy—Dominick knew he had to tell his parents too.

Gene Crow worked on Sunday afternoons, so Dominick always made his weekly phone call home during that time. Like clockwork, Crow would tape an itemized list of his calls with a total owed, to his blanket-door on the fifth of every month, with a handwritten note that said, "Due IMMEDIATELY." When it came to matters of money owed, Crow did not muck about.

The third Sunday in April, Dominick called home. Connie answered the phone, and after hearing the rundown on her high school happenings, Laura came on.

"Mom, I've got something to tell you."

"How bad is it? Are you in jail?"

"No, Mom, I'm not, but thanks for believing in me." They both chuckled, then Dominick said, "I met someone."

"Of course you did."

"I ... what?"

"Of course you've met someone. Why else would you stay somewhere like that for so long? Wisconsin isn't really the garden spot of the United States, especially over the winter. Your Dad and I have just been wondering when you were going to tell us."

"But—no, Mom, we've only been together for a month."

"You've only known her for a month?"

"Well, no. I met her right after I got here."

"Mmm-hmm."

"You always have the knack for confusing me."

"That's because a mother always knows the truth. I know what you're going to tell me before you even pick up the phone. So, when do we meet her? Are you bringing her home?"

"No way, Mom. We've only been dating a month. I'm not about to ask her to set out on a cross-country drive with me."

Laura changed the subject, talking about how Sam's apprenticeship was progressing and how people were so disappointed that they couldn't bring their lawn mowers by for repair any more.

Dominick's mind lingered on the idea, though. An image of he and Emily, riding in the Chevelle with the windows down and the music up, ran through his mind time and again.

That same night, sitting on the bed in Emily's room, waiting for Melody and Sandy to stop by, he broached the subject.

"So, I called my folks today."

"Yeah? All good?"

"Yeah. They don't like it when I'm gone so long. They're trying to get me to come home, at least for a visit."

Emily reached out and took his hand. "I don't love the sound of that, but I understand. So, you going?"

Dominick scooched closer. "How about you come with me?"

"What, to California?"

"Yes. If we don't stop to gawk, it's only a two day drive. We could take two days driving out there, stay a few days, so my folks are happy, then two days back. They'll put my sister on the couch, you can have her room, and I'll be just on the other side of the wall, with my brother. You'll be out of school for the summer pretty quick, we could do it then."

Emily leaned back against the wall, contemplating. A long moment later, she said, "No. How long have we been dating? Not long enough to set out on a trip like that together."

"I figured you were going to say your parents wouldn't like it."

"They wouldn't like it, that's right, but I make my own decisions."

I love you so, Emily, but sometimes I wish you weren't so perfectly yourself. So damned level-headed.

Dominick dropped it, but the image of them driving fast over the open road with a warm wind blowing in their hair, didn't dissipate easily.

ONE WARM LATE-SPRING evening, after they'd been together several months, Dominick and Emily sat on a blanket in Deland Park, looking out at Lake Michigan. More accurately, Emily sat on a blanket. Dominick stretched out in front of her, with his head in her lap.

Emily was telling Dominick about one of her strange dreams, where she was on a beach, getting what she called a moon-tan. "It was so crystal-clear real. There were half a dozen moons in the sky, and their rays were like a spiritual cleansing. Pretty weird, right?"

"No weirder than any of your other dreams. I think you have a future as a writer."

Emily was running her fingers through his tangle of curls. She changed the subject. Quietly, she said, "You are a most unusual boy, Dominick Davidner."

"You don't know the half of it, but what do you mean in particular?"

"Well, we've been dating for months now, and you've never pushed me about sex. Believe me, that makes you a most unusual boy."

Emily, I love you every way possible. Of course I want you like that, but this is so complicated. And, we're young. We've got a lifetime ahead.

"It gets weirder. I'm a virgin."

Emily giggled, which made her look even younger. "I think I knew that part of the puzzle. Don't ask me how."

"I love you, Emily."

Her eyes widened. "Oh."

Damnit. Too soon. I knew it.

He shrugged. "Don't worry about it. I know it's quick. I can't say I always fall in love fast, because I've never loved anyone else like I do you, Emily. But, it's okay, no pressure."

"Right. My boyfriend just told me he loved me out of the blue, but no pressure. I love you too, Dominick, I just wasn't quite ready to tell you that yet." She leaned over and kissed his upside down lips, long and slow.

They stayed in the park until the warmth had left the air and they had to wrap up in the blanket. Neither of them wanted to leave the sweetness of the moment. Even as dark descended, they stayed, watching the play of the lights on the water of the lake.

In full dark, they finally gave up, folded up their blanket, and walked hand in hand back to the Chevelle. Way too soon for either of them, they arrived back at Emily's.

"Good things come to those who wait, Nicky," she said, and jumped out of the car and ran into her house.

Dominick drove home slowly, meandering along, letting his mind drift. Eventually, he pulled into his regular parking spot and let himself in through the side door. In his room, he didn't even turn on the light, just stripped down to his boxers and slipped into bed.

He laid there for a long time, tossing one way, then turning the other. His brain was filled with Emily, and sleep would not come. After an hour, he was ready to turn on the light and just read until he couldn't hold his eyes open any longer, when he heard a tapping at the window above his bed.

He bolted upright. Listened intently, and heard it again. He kneeled on the bed, unlatched the window, and it slid open all the way. Emily tumbled through the window and fell head-first onto the bed before tumbling onto the floor, where she collapsed in a fit of giggles.

Dominick scooped her up, helping her onto the bed. Before he could say anything, she put a finger against his lips.

She stood, grace restored, and pushed the sundress she was wearing off her shoulders and let it fall to the ground. Moonlight through the window silhouetted her. Dominick let out an involuntary sigh. She pushed him back against his pillow, then climbed under the covers with him.

"It's cold in here. Keep me warm."

Later, Emily reached up to touch Dominick's face in the dark. It was wet with silent tears.

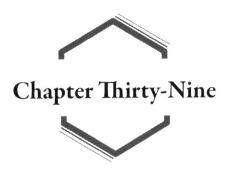

Chapter Thirty-Nine

No one ever saw a rainbow without a little rain, and even in the summer of Dominick's greatest contentment, there was the occasional thunderhead. He and Emily were perfectly compatible, as he had known they would be, because they already had been. They liked much of the same music, movies, books, and people. Even more importantly, they disliked most of the same things.

The only area they ever fell into disagreement was when Dominick wanted to go rushing headlong into the future, blazing a trail that Emily was not yet ready to walk down. Dominick was not a jealous man, and he trusted Emily completely. Still, he managed to goof up from time to time.

On the 4th of July, a whole group of friends gathered at the park to blow off steam before the summer evaporated when they weren't looking.

It wasn't just the tried and true foursome of Dominick, Emily, Melody, and Sandy, but another half dozen friends the girls knew at the UW. They took over two of the picnic tables at the park and spread out pizzas, chips, and of course, illicit beer and cheap wine. One of the other men at the gathering was a dark-haired boy named Felix who seemed to know Emily very well. When she first saw him, she ran up to him and threw her arms around him, then brought him over to introduce him to Dominick.

Felix shook Dominick's hand, and said, "You, my friend, are a lucky man."

You know, I already know that, and I don't really need you pointing it out.

Someone brought a Frisbee, someone else had brought some grass, and after an hour or so, everyone had loosened up and was laughing and telling stories about classes and college professors who, of course, Dominick did not know. He did his best to stay involved in the conversation, but his mind wandered.

It will be better when our frames of reference catch up to each other, and we all know the same people, and have some history behind us, instead of having it all in front of us.

Dominick threw the Frisbee around with a guy named Bruce, and worked up a sweat. When he came back, looking for something to wipe his face off, Emily was sitting on Felix's lap on the bench, surrounded by other friends.

She smiled at Dominick, and reached a hand out so he could help her up. "Having fun, baby?"

Dominick just stood looking at her, then looking at Felix, who seemed to be enjoying his discomfort. Instead of helping Emily up, he ignored her smile, her hand, her greeting, and turned and walked down toward the lake.

Emily let him pout by himself for quite some time, but eventually came down. She was no longer smiling.

"What the hell is wrong with you?"

Dominick shrugged and looked out over the water.

"If you want to tell me that you're having some sort of a medical emergency, and came down here to die alone, that's fine. If you want to tell me that you're jealous of me hanging out with friends I have known for a long time, we need to have a serious conversation."

Uh-oh.

"It was just kind of a shock to walk up and find you sitting on someone else's lap."

Emily nodded as if she understood completely.

Uh-oh again.

"Oh, sure I get it. Your girlfriend, who you *own*, was showing affection to another man. Who wouldn't get upset by that?"

I forgot how sarcastic she gets when she's pissed off. How did I used to cool her down?

"It's not like that, Em." Dominick reached out for her hand, which she jerked away.

Not like that, obviously.

"Okay then, Dominick, tell me what it is like? When you come up to me, and I smile and reach for you, and you turn your back away and storm off, what exactly is it like?"

It's like I screwed up. It's like I saw you with another man and lost my mind for a minute. Wait. Why not just tell her that?

"Okay. You're right. I saw you sitting on another guy's lap, and it killed me. You know me. I'm not the jealous type. But it hurt more than I can probably admit. I walked away to cool off."

"And what's that message to me? When I do something that pushes your buttons, you're just gonna storm off and leave me alone to figure it out?"

"No," Dominick said, as if to himself. He looked Emily in the eye. "No. I messed up, Em. I've felt like I was on the outside looking in all day, like everybody knew everybody but me, and I let it get to me." He reached out, put a hand on her shoulder. She didn't pull away. "I'm sorry. I'm an idiot."

Emily tilted her head to one side.

She always seems to be looking right through me when she does that.

"You're not an idiot. Sometimes you just act like one. Most of the time, you're a pretty cool guy. That's why I'm with you, you know?"

Dominick nodded, reached down, grabbed her hand and kissed it.

"Come on," she said. "The pizza's cold, but it's still good. Somebody rolled a bunch of joints, so the food will all be gone soon."

They held hands on the way back to the picnic.

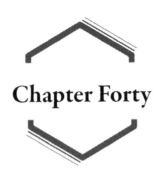

Chapter Forty

A month later, Dominick drove to Emily's house. She had phoned him earlier that day—which brought on a warning from Gene Crow—and asked him to come over. When he pulled up, he saw that Melody's car was already parked in the driveway.

Just as he stepped up onto the porch, the door swung open, as if by a ghost?

"Umm... Hello?" Dominick said.

The only answer was a giggle from behind the door.

"Ah, it is the ghost of Melody, dearly departed all these years gone by."

Dominick pushed against the door a little and heard an "Oof" from the other side. "Pretty corporal for a ghost, though."

"Smart ass," Melody said, pushing her way out. "Everybody loves a little ass, but nobody loves a smart ass."

"Duly noted," Dominick said, following her down the hall to Emily's room.

Inside, Sandy and Emily were sitting on the bed, surrounded by papers.

"Did I suddenly time travel?" Dominick asked. "That looks a lot like school work."

"Well, yes and no," Emily said, seriously. "It's my application for UW-Madison."

"Ho—hold on. You said you were going there for your third and fourth year."

"I know I did. But, when I was registering for classes at UW-Sheboygan, what they had to offer was just so limited that I went in and got a catalog for Madison. What they offer there is amazing. Everything I want. So, I'm thinking of going there a year early. Then, I can finish my prerequisites, but I can also start taking some of the classes I really want to take."

Dominick plopped down into the bean bag chair.

"I don't even know if I'll get in."

"Of course, you'll get in, Em. Has there ever been anything you've gone after that you haven't got?"

"I never got that pony I asked for every year."

"I would hate you being so far away." Dominick tried not to sound like a pouty child, but failed.

"It's only two hours. I'm going to go up and find off-campus housing, so you can come up and visit, and sometimes I'll drive down just to snuggle in your blanket fort.

"What about the cost?"

I've been working at the insurance company part time all year. They gave me full-time hours over the summer. I've got enough saved up to get me started. Plus, once Mom and Dad saw that I was really serious about this, they agreed to pay part of the cost of housing, too."

That's what I mean, Emily. You are an unstoppable force. Once you set your sights on something, you're going to find a way to make it happen. So, why am I fighting it? This is a long game, so if I need to be patient for a while, I will. Or, hell, there's nothing holding me here. I can get a gas station job in Madison just as easily as I did here. Might not be able to find another apartment where the walls are made out of old wool blankets, though.

Dominick stood up, wiggled his way in between Emily and Sandy, and took her into his arms. "You're right. You're right, of course. I should just get a tattoo that says, 'Emily's right,' that you can point at when I am tempted to disagree with you."

"That would be a very good idea, except for, ick, tattoos."

Just shows you can be wrong sometimes, too, Em.

A FEW WEEKS LATER, Emily got the expected news—that she was part of the last group to be accepted into the University of Wisconsin-Madison for the fall semester of 1978. She didn't want to wait until the last minute to secure her housing, so she, Sandy, and Dominick made the drive to Madison.

She found a great house—no creepy landlord, actual walls in her bedroom—immediately. *See,* her eyes said, looking at Dominick, *everything is falling into place.*

Dominick hadn't told Emily, but he had already given his notice at the gas station, and he tucked the phone numbers for several other rooms for rent numbers in the back of his jeans pocket so he could call them when he got home.

Whither thou goest, and all that stuff, Em.

Class was scheduled to start on September 25th, but Emily wanted to go up a week early, so she could familiarize herself with the town and the campus. They made a caravan going down to Madison—Emily's little Pinto, Dominick's Chevelle, and Melody once again driving her dad's Bronco. She only had a single room in a boarding house, but she had her desk, and lamps, and quilts, and her artwork and an electric pot to heat water in, and her record player and boxes of other miscellaneous stuff that she just knew she couldn't survive without.

Within an hour of walking through the door, her bedroom looked almost like an exact replica of her room back in Sheboygan, minus the Andy Gibb and Shaun Cassidy posters she had outgrown.

Sandy and Melody said goodbye first, making an excuse to get out and let Dominick and Emily spend a few minutes alone.

Dominick held her tight against him.

Why do I have this irrational fear that I am going to lose her? I know she loves me. I know what kind of person she is, but there it is, anyway. I need to get it together. I am a fifty year old man. I've gotta grow up.

"Enjoy your new digs, Em. I know you'll need to get a few weeks to get settled in, then I'll drive up and see you."

"Yes, sounds perfect. It means a lot to me that you're able to give me the space I need, Nicky. I love you."

"Love you, too." He held her face in his hands, kissed her softly, and let himself out of her room.

On the way out of Madison, he stopped and looked at a few different rooms that were for rent. None of them had the charm of the blanket fort, but they also all had blessedly normal landlords, not creeper overlords who thought their houses were their own fiefdoms.

My only regret is that I'll never make the Mantle of Fame.

The last one he looked at was a bit farther away from the UW, and so was also a bit cheaper. He put down the first month's rent, and told the landlord he'd be back to move in soon.

With a light heart, convinced he was doing the right thing, he told Gene Crow that he would be moving out at the end of September.

Everything is falling into place.

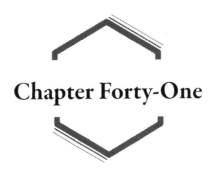

Chapter Forty-One

There is a certain irony in the fact that, quite often, just as we believe everything is falling into place, everything has already begun to fall apart. And so it was for Dominick Davidner.

He put in his two weeks at the service station, gathered up his few items from the Crow Manse—no more, really, than he had packed in the day he had arrived—and drove to Madison. He stopped at a small jewelry store in a strip mall on the outskirts of town and made a purchase, then went straight to his new room, unpacked his clothes and his books, and cast about for something to do.

Feels strange to be here, just a few minutes away from Emily, and not being with her. I know she needs her space, though.

Dominick invested his time in going around town and putting in job applications at gas stations, garages, and car dealerships—anywhere that needed someone who could work on engines. After half a dozen stops, nothing looked promising.

Gonna need to find something pretty quick. The savings account is dwindling. In those time travel movies, they always make it easy—go bet on a big sporting event, or buy a stock that's gonna skyrocket. Problem is, I was never much of a sports fan, and I don't have the sports almanac that Michael J. Fox did. I have no idea what stock to invest in, circa 1978, either. I guess Microsoft will be a great investment when it goes public, but I'm not even sure when that is. I guess I should have paid more attention to these things.

Finally, Dominick had waited until he could wait no more. He drove to Emily's new place, knocked on the door, and asked for her. When she appeared at the front door, she smiled and was happy to see him. She led him upstairs to her room. She had obviously been studying, as a book was open on the desk, and a small, goose-necked desk lamp was turned on.

Dominick took the scene in, then said, "Studying, huh?"

"Yes, Sherlock. What was your first clue? The fact that I'm a college student, or the pile of textbooks open on my desk?"

He smiled. "Funny girl. You are such a funny girl."

Dominick lifted Emily off the ground and backed her up until he dropped her on the bed. He kneeled down on both knees in front of her and put his head in her lap.

"I've missed you, Em."

"Missed you, too, Nicky. It will be a little crazy for a while. My course load is a lot heavier now, which means a lot more studying, plus I've got to find a part time job waitressing or something. But, it will settle down soon enough. We'll figure it out."

"I've had a lot of time to think about things, these past few weeks, and I want to tell you part of what I've figured out."

"Okay," she said, stroking his face. "Or, we could always, you know ..." she jerked her head toward the fluffy pillows at the head of the bed.

"Yes, that would be good, too, but I really want to tell you this."

She smirked. "Must be pretty damn important for you to pass up such a good offer. Okay, fine. I'm listening."

"I really hated being apart from you. I wandered around town, kinda lost. I hung out with Mel and Sandy a little, but it's not the same without you there."

"That's because I am so wonderful." Emily giggled, and ran her hands up under his shirt.

Dominick pushed them down.

"You are trying to distract me, but I am strong." Dominick smiled, the smile that always made Emily want to jump on him.

He grew serious. "I have to tell you. I quit my job at the station."

Emily looked puzzled. "Why?"

Dominick held a hand up. "Also, I gave my notice to Gene Crow and moved out."

"What? Where are you going? Are you moving back to California?"

"Em, I could never leave you. I moved up here. I've got a room about two miles from here."

"Oh." That single syllable that Emily used for so many purposes. "Oh."

Dominick got halfway up, fished in his pocket for a little blue box and got back down on one knee in front of Emily. Her hand flew to her mouth.

"Oh!"

Dominick opened the small box. There was a ring was inside. It was a diamond ring in the same way a Hot Wheels is a car.

Emily's eyes filled with tears, spilled over, and ran down her face.

Tears are good. Come on, Emily, just say 'Yes,' and the rest of our life is set.

Instead, she shook her head, and said, "You just don't listen to me, Dominick."

Dominick was stunned, and rocked back on his heels. His mouth dropped open.

She sniffed back more tears, and said, "You really don't listen," as if he hadn't been listening the first time she said it. "Why did I break up with Burke? Because he was moving us along too fast, and I wasn't ready for it, so I let him go. That was less than six months ago. Do you think my life has changed that much in just six months?"

Dominick shut his mouth, closed the box, and slipped it back into his pocket.

Emily swiped the tears away from her eyes. "Oh, Dominick, I really do love you. You're so special to me, but I can't do this anymore."

"Em, I'm sorry. I thought this was a good thing. I just want us to be together."

Emily shook her head so violently that one of her tears flew off and landed on Dominick's cheek. He reached up and touched it gently.

"I can't do this anymore. It all hurts too much. First, Burke, now you. I need to just be alone."

"Wait. What?" Dominick froze. "What are you saying?" He tasted a coppery fear in his mouth.

Emily wiped more tears away, calm now. "I'm saying, 'No, Dominick, I won't marry you.' I'm nineteen years old. I don't even know who I am yet—"

"You know who you are better than anyone I've ever met, Emily."

"—and I don't know when I will know. I was afraid of this from the beginning. I knew better. Melody told me that you had been following us around, before you 'accidentally' met us at the bowling alley. I really should have known better, but I liked you Dominick, and eventually, I loved you. But, now I see." Even quieter, she said, "Now I know." She shook her head. "No more. I'm so sorry, Dominick, but I just can't do it."

Dominick sat down flat on her floor. Now, his own tears were coming, hot and fast.

"Wait, Em. I get it now. I do. Let's just forget this happened. I'll give up my place here and move back to Sheboygan. Whatever it takes. Please, just don't say we're done."

She shook her head.

Dominick came to a snap decision.

"I can't believe I'm going to tell you this, Em, but I feel like I have to. This isn't our first lifetime together."

Emily winced as though she was in pain. "What?"

Dominick kept his voice calm. If his story was going to be insane, he wanted to sound as rational as he could.

"We've known each other before. In another lifetime. We were married, and we were happy." Dominick laughed bitterly. "We were both teachers. We owned a little house with a white picket fence around it, as cliché as that sounds. It's so hard that you don't you remember any of this."

Emily's hand was at her mouth again. She shook her head and began to back away.

"And then ... and then, I was killed, and I woke up back in my nine year old body."

"Dominick, stop!"

"Please, just let me finish. It's important."

Emily edged toward her desk. She put her hand on her pink princess phone.

Dominick spoke louder and faster. "Everything I've done since I opened my eyes back here was to try and give us a chance to find what we already had—our life together."

Emily took the phone out of the cradle, and when she spoke, a note of hysteria crept into her voice. "You don't get it. There is no 'we' anymore. We're done. I can't take this craziness any more. I don't want to see you again, Dominick. Get out, or I'm going to call the police."

Dominick took one step toward her, but Emily flinched away in fear.

Dominick froze. *Oh my God, what have I done? She's afraid of me.* He turned and ran from her room.

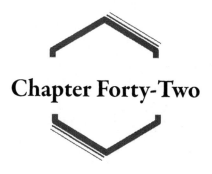

Chapter Forty-Two

Dominick stumbled out of Emily's room, and down the stairs. He passed one of her roommates before he got to the front door. She stared at him, open mouthed, but he didn't care. He climbed into his car and started it. The low rumble, the menacing growl, was there, but he didn't hear it. His blood was pounding in his ears.

He slowly leaned forward and laid his head against the steering wheel. Tears dripped off his face and into his lap. Numbly, he shifted into drive and pulled away from the curb. He had no destination. He felt as though he might never have another destination ever again.

He drove through Madison and got on a highway headed west.

Okay. I blew it. She's right. I wasn't paying attention. I was so single-mindedly focused on recreating what we had, that I didn't read the situation right in front of me. This would have been fine for me. I'm a middle-aged man, but she's not. She's a young girl. She needs to live.

Dominick drove blindly, only keeping the car on the road and in his lane subconsciously.

She'll change her mind, though. Right?

He thought back to the stricken look on Emily's face when he had pulled out the ring. Or worse, the fear on her face when he had stepped toward her.

No. She won't. Time to stop fooling myself. That's what got me into this mess. So, what now, then?

Dominick drove blindly on, mile after mile, until darkness fell. He reached down and turned his headlights on. His gas tank still read half full. He pushed on, doing his best to blank everything from his mind, failing time and again

Up ahead, the road curved to the left, then onto a bridge that crossed a river, maybe fifty feet below. He pushed down on the accelerator. His speed ticked up to 65, 70, 75. The growl of the engine increased in volume and pitch.

When the road turned left, Dominick held the Chevelle in a straight line. The tires left the pavement, hit dirt and gravel, shimmied a little, but held their trajectory.

A moment later, the car shot off the embankment and all four wheels left the ground. Dominick never took his foot off the accelerator, even when the RPMs went above the redline.

The headlights cut through the darkness at a sharply downward angle, reflecting the gray water below. The car hit the water nose first, slamming Dominick into the steering wheel and windshield with horrific force.

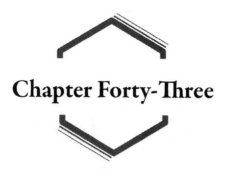

Chapter Forty-Three

"Oh. Dominick, no," Carrie said. "That's not the answer. That's never the answer!"

Carrie had killed herself a dozen times when she was on Earth, doing exactly what Dominick was doing: resetting, hoping for a better result. The irony of scolding Dominick for the same thing she had done so many times did not occur to her.

She spoke so vehemently that Maruna actually took her eyes off her pyxis for a moment.

"Sorry," Carrie mumbled, then returned her attention to the car driving off a cliff and plunging into a river. She backed it up, let it roll forward, backed it up, let it roll forward. After she did that half a dozen times, she saw that nothing was changing. As she had done when Dominick had nearly killed Mr. Bratski, she reached into the image and pinched a bit of it away.

It played out the same.

She pinched out more, and more, and more, but the scene never changed. Each time, the car left the road, jumped down the embankment, and Dominick was recycled.

She was so focused on trying to change what was happening, that she didn't notice both Bertellia and Margenta, standing over her shoulder watching her.

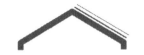

Chapter Forty-Four
Dimension AG54298-M25736
1968

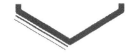

D ominick opened his eyes with a gasp. He was staring into Connie's brown eyes.

Her lower lip trembled. "Bubby okay?"

Dominick let his head fall back onto the carpet with a thud and sighed.

I've got to start thinking things through.

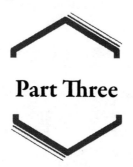

Part Three

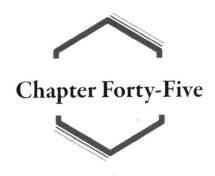

Chapter Forty-Five

The next ten years were not easy for Dominick. When he woke up back in his nine year old body again, he felt overwhelming anger toward Emily.

I thought we were soul mates, but no soul mate would ever act that way. And, *I thought we were meant to be, but I must have been wrong.* And, *I thought you would always love me, no matter what.*

Time, as it almost always does, brought perspective. When he was away from her intoxicating presence, he was able to see that year he spent in Sheboygan more clearly. He saw the clarity of the messages Emily had been sending him, and he finally got perspective on what his actions had looked like to her.

And now, here I am again, a fifty year old man who acted like a teenager, stuck in the body of a nine year old boy.

He was a more veteran time traveler this time around, though, and he knew what to expect. He didn't fight back and bloody Sam's nose. He and his friends never even ran into Billy Stitts while they were walking around town, so he never hurt him and put him into the hospital. He did encourage his dad to work on the Dodge Town out in the garage, but he just did that to have something to do, and to clear out room for the small engine repair that he knew he and his dad would start again.

Even though they got the Dodge on the road, he was never tempted to take it for a joyride, and so he never killed Mr. Bratski's roses, or, very nearly, Mr. Bratski himself. He did remember Mr. and

Mrs. Bratski kindly from his previous life, though, and mowed their lawn for free every summer.

The ten years that it took to get back to where he had been before he drove his car into the lake dragged inexorably. His second pass through that decade had held the attraction of nostalgia, but that evaporated on a third trip through. Even the thrill of seeing his family again was muted by knowing that he had essentially handed himself a ten year prison sentence, just to get back to where he had been.

He was a quieter, less boisterous boy this trip through his life. He had begun to feel, to a certain extent, that his life's energy was ebbing. He used the many long hours to turn the year he had spent in Wisconsin over and over in his mind. The more he compared those months with Emily to the happy years they had spent as husband and wife, the clearer it became. He had gambled everything on the innate attraction that he felt toward Emily, and the fact that she would feel it to the same extent, no matter that the circumstances were so different from their initial meeting.

In his first life, Dominick and Emily had met when he had left his job teaching in Oakland and accepted the position in Middle Falls. They were both in their late twenties and ready to look for a life partner.

In Sheboygan, Dominick had done everything he could to cut in line and get ahead of the game. Meanwhile, Emily, gently at first, finally with force, had told him she wasn't ready. He could see that clearly now, but with that clarity, came a new problem. If it had seemed an eternity to wait until he had graduated from high school, it would be even worse to try and wait until they had met organically. That meant a nine year slog through elementary, junior high, and high school, then four years of college, and he would still have to wait another four or five years to meet her again. It felt like an eternity stretching out in front of him.

But the pain of Emily's rejection was still fresh in his mind and heart, despite the years he had now spent in this third life. So he was resolved to keep his head down, pass the time as best he could, and be prepared for the chance to rebuild the bridge to Emily properly when the time came.

And as it always does, the time passed.

Those early years, he was limited by his age and size, and he watched the same television shows with his family, fixed the same lawnmower engines, and generally treaded water.

He got the same good grades he had gotten previously, and graduated again with a 3.93 GPA. He could have gotten a 4.0, but he didn't want to attract attention to himself, and take that honor away from someone else who deserved it. His only real goal was to get good enough grades and participate in enough activities that he could get some scholarships and get accepted into Cabrillo College in Santa Cruz.

Of course, in this life, he didn't make the drive north to watch The Turtles graduate from Hartfield Academy. If he had shown up, no one there would have known him. Dying and living again multiple times had shown him the transiency of relationships, if nothing else.

He spent the summer after graduating high school fixing lawnmowers and saving his money. Even with his scholarships, college was going to be expensive.

Through it all, the boredom and the repetitiveness, Emily never left his mind or his heart. Even though he had no intention on setting off across the country to see her, he still felt the strong need to make sure she was still there.

He subscribed to the Sheboygan *Depression* early in his junior year and read each new issue cover to cover, even though the news was almost a week old by the time it reached him. That didn't matter.

He just scanned for any mention of Emily's name. In two years of reading it, he had never seen it.

On the Fourth of July, while Laura was cooking fried chicken and making potato salad for an outdoor supper before the fireworks, Dominick slipped away from the house.

He had not bought the same Chevelle this life. He associated it too much with the life he had just lived. Instead, he bought a more practical 1971 Ford pickup. It wasn't beautiful—in fact, he called it *The Ugly Truckling*—but it was a lot easier to haul lawn mowers and Evinrude motors around in it.

Dominick started the truck and reversed out onto the street in front of the house. He didn't go far, just a few blocks down to the convenience store, and the payphone outside. He had thought of making this phone call for months—years, really, if he was honest with himself—but like every other major decision in his life, he was impetuous and did it on the spur of the moment.

He stepped into the payphone and swung the door closed behind him, but it was immediately stultifying, and the enclosed space and heat made it smell suspiciously of urine. He swung the door open again and let the fresh air in. He reached in his pocket and scooped out a handful of quarters. He dropped them on the steel counter, then stacked them into piles of four.

From memory, he dialed the number he had memorized in Sheboygan the year before.

Not going to talk to her. I just need to hear her voice. Know that she's okay.

An operator came on the line and said, "One dollar and seventy five cents, for the first three minutes, please."

Dominick dropped seven of his quarters into the slot. There was a distant, tinny buzzing on the other end of the line. It rang three, four, five times.

Nobody home. Okay.

He reached to pick up the rest of his quarters.

He heard a noisy click on the other end of the line. A woman's voice said, "Hello?"

Dominick's throat grew tight. Sweating in the heat of the summer day, the phone grew slippery in his hand. He cleared his throat, and said, "Is Emily there?"

There was a long pause, then the woman's voice said, mechanically, "Who is this?"

Dominick was ready for that question. "Brad Stevens," he said, giving her the most anonymous name he could think of this side of John Smith.

"How did you know Emily?"

Dominick was nervous, and the past tense slipped right by him, unnoticed.

"I'm just a friend, from school."

"I see. Mr. Stevens, Emily passed away almost five years ago."

Dominick stood dead still, the phone still in his hands, but he wasn't hearing. Her words echoed through his head, tearing paths like a bullet.

"Mr. Stevens? Mr. Stevens, are you there?" Her voice, more distant, as if she had turned her head away from the receiver, said, "He said he was a friend from school."

A moment later, a man's stern voice came on the line. "Hello? When did you know Emily? Hello?"

The phone slipped from Dominick's grasp and hung at the end of its braided metal cord, swaying back and forth.

Dominick stumbled from the phone booth, leaving the stacks of quarters behind. He made it to his pickup, then reached one hand out to steady himself. His world spun around him, and he slumped to the ground with his head resting against the front bumper.

An unknowable time later, he started the truck and pulled out of the parking lot. He drove without thinking. He passed the city limits sign for Emeryville and kept driving west. The further he drove, the faster he went. A few miles out of town, the road curved left. To the right was a steep hillside, covered by rocks, trees and underbrush. Dominick floored the accelerator.

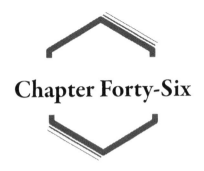

Chapter Forty-Six

Margenta grasped Carrie's pyxis roughly.

"Aaaack!" Carrie yelped in surprise. She had been so focused on undoing Dominick's suicide that she hadn't known she was being observed.

Margenta pulled the pyxis from Carrie's hands and slipped it into a fold in her billowing white robe.

"You have already been warned. Now you will face the Council." Margenta put one hand on Bertellia's shoulder and another on Carrie's.

The scene shifted as though someone had changed the channel. The three of them were in a room so large, it might have been outdoors, if not for walls in the far distance and an arching ceiling that rose as far as the eye could see.

The three of them stood on an inky-black floor. Hovering in front of them were seven desks. Bertellia leaned over to Carrie and whispered, "This is the Temporal Relocation High Council."

Margenta shot a look at Bertellia, and Bertellia hushed, then took a step back.

There were seven figures, one standing at each of the desks. They appeared to wear robes made entirely of light, which made it difficult to focus on, or even see, their faces.

Carrie's eyes widened. *I didn't think there was much they could do to me, other than maybe tell me I couldn't do this job any more, but this place, those ... beings are unsettling.*

The being in the middle desk, dressed in a shimmering robe the color of the sky at sunset, raised her hand and said, "Margenta, why have you asked the council to convene?"

Carrie shook her head slightly. She wasn't sure if the voice—which sounded as melodic as a brook babbling across stones—was heard through her ears, or just through her mind.

Margenta bowed her head reverently. "Blessed One, one of my Watchers has deviated from her duties of feeding the Machine. Instead of performing her only task, she becomes involved," she sniffed a bit, "in the outcomes of their lives."

"This is against our protocol."

"Yes. Thus, my request for the meeting of the High Council."

"Watcher, what is your name?"

"Carrie."

"Is what Margenta says true? Are you interfering with the lives of humans on Earth?"

"Yes," Carrie said, trying to take the shake out of her voice. "It is."

"Why?"

"Because I refuse to watch my humans suffer needlessly."

"You understand that they cannot actually be harmed?"

"Yes, but their psyches can be harmed. I don't like to see them in pain."

An odd buzzing sound emanated from the beings behind the desks as they conferred.

"Do you understand that this emotional pain feeds the Machine?"

"Yes, but so does any emotion. I would rather gather happiness, contentment, joy."

The being behind the far right hand desk, who wore a robe the color of shifting sands, said, "But, do you understand that the emotional pain you witness is likely part of their growth process?"

Carrie considered this, then quietly said, "No, I don't. I don't interfere often. Pain is everywhere. I just do my best to mitigate it for those I watch over."

"Margenta, what do you recommend we do?"

"I recommend reassignment or recycling. Perhaps another few passes through lives on Earth will bring her the needed perspective."

The blue-robed being in the middle desk said, "Thank you, Margenta, for bringing this to our attention. We will pass judgement now." The odd buzzing, rising and falling in pitch and harmonics, recommenced for several seconds.

"It is the judgement of the Council that ..."

A breeze riffled the air, carrying the scent of a faraway dream. The room became brighter, but there was no apparent source for the light.

Carrie sucked in her breath. Her whole body tingled. A calm settled over her that she had never known.

"Oh!" Blue-Robe said. "We are honored by Your presence." She bowed her head.

Carrie looked around to see who, or what she was referring to, but saw nothing else. She listened intently, but could not hear a voice.

After a moment of silence, Blue-Robe said, "I see. Yes, of course. As You wish."

The light faded. The breeze dissipated. The sense of calm belonging that had washed over Carrie slowly receded.

There was a great sigh that spread across those assembled, as if the connection that had brought them all together, was now broken.

"The ruling of the Council has ... evolved. There will be a new protocol in place, effective immediately. The IS That IS has conveyed that what has been in the past will no longer be. The IS That IS has spoken. The word for this new protocol will be, *kindness*. The IS That

IS wishes us to retrain ourselves to learn kindness and compassion for those we watch over."

The buzzing, in a lower key this time, recommenced.

"Margenta, Bertellia, as part of the training program, you will be reassigned as Watchers. Carrie, you will be Watcher Superior now, and will be in charge of training."

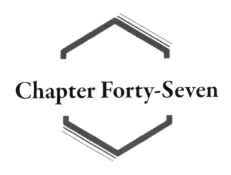

Chapter Forty-Seven

At the last possible moment, Dominick let off the gas and braked hard. The truck had veered onto the shoulder and fishtailed on the loose gravel, ending up sideways, with the back end resting on dirt.

I promised myself I would think things through. Stop doing shit without thinking. But, what is there to think about? Emily is gone from this world. No matter what I do, no matter how long I wait, she will never be here.

Dominick looked up and noticed his surroundings for the first time. He checked for oncoming traffic, turned the wheel and drove back the way he came.

What are my choices? Kill myself again, start over again, and hope that Emily is still there next time? I might go even crazier than I am if I have to live through this again. But, if I just stay here, then what? Just resign myself to a life without Emily? What does that look like? Wait and eventually meet someone else I can love, even though I know they would always be second in my heart to Em?

Dominick did his best to gather his wits about him and drove home. He parked in his normal spot and walked in the house. As soon as Laura saw him, she said, "Nicky! What's wrong?"

"Huh? Nothing, Mom, why?"

"You look like you've seen a ghost!"

I'm the only ghost around here, Mom.

She hurried over to him and laid the back of her hand against first his flushed cheek, then his forehead.

"You don't have a fever. Come on, sit down over here on the couch."

"Ah, thanks, I'm really not feeling well. I think I'll go lay down on my bed for a little while."

"Good idea. I'll have dinner ready soon enough. If you fall asleep, you just rest, and I'll save you a plate."

Dominick lay down in the darkened bedroom he shared with Sam and did his best to think, but his thoughts just chased each other round and round.

No matter what, it comes down to two choices. Go on, and live without Emily, or start over again, and have a chance to be with her.

He followed those dueling ideas around, like water circling the drain. Soon, he was asleep, and dreamed of Emily, as he so often did. Typically, when he dreamed of her, she was far away, and he tried to reach her but his muscles turned to jelly, or flat ground grew so steep he couldn't climb to her.

Today, though, she was near him. He reached out to her and said, "Em, what am I supposed to do?" She didn't speak, but reached for him, touching his face. He reached up for her hand, but opened his eyes to see his mother.

"Just wanted to check on you, Nicky. You've been asleep for hours, honey. How are you feeling?"

Suicidal, if you want to know the truth.

"I'm fine, Mom. Just got a little bug or something, I think."

"Why don't you come outside? I saved you some fried chicken, and your dad's getting ready to cut up a watermelon."

Dominick nodded, stood up and slipped his shoes on. He felt strange, like he was wrapped in gauze and walking through a cloud.

He wandered out to the picnic table they had set up in the front yard. The sun had slipped behind the horizon and he could see a few stars beginning to twinkle in the sky.

"There he is!" Joe said. "Ready for watermelon?"

"Sure," Dominick said, although he had never been less hungry in his life.

Joe sliced a piece and set it in front of him.

Neighborhood kids ran down the street with sparklers, making crazy designs in the air.

Dominick sat and stared out at them, at the sky, at the deepening gloom. He didn't notice it, but tears had formed and slipped down his cheeks.

Laura gave Joe an alarmed look but stayed calm. She laid her hand on Dominick's shoulder and said "Come on honey, let's get you back in bed."

As soon as he lay down again, Dominick slipped into a deep, dreamless sleep.

When he woke up in the morning, the fog of the previous day had cleared. He awoke before the sun was up, and already had the coffee on when Joe came out of the bedroom to get ready for work.

"Hi, Dad," he said, as he poured two cups, black.

"Hey," Joe said, blowing the steam off his cup. He looked appraisingly at Dominick. "Feeling better?"

Dominick smiled. "Yeah, better. Thanks, Dad."

"Good boy. Thanks for the cup." He collected his lunch box and was off to work. Dominick went out to the little one-car garage where he had worked on engines both large and small for almost twenty years, spread over two lifetimes. He lifted and moved several of the motors and mowers that he had been working on over the previous few days, making space.

While he was doing that, Laura got in her car to go to work as well. She gave him a smile and a wave.

Dominick got in his truck, drove it into the garage and shut the door behind him. Working steadily, he picked up the shop rags he kept stacked in the corner and filled all the holes and cracks in the little garage as best he could. He turned the little transistor radio to the same country station it always played, then started the truck and laid down across the bench seat,

One more try, Emily. One more try.

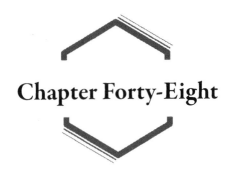

Chapter Forty-Eight

Carrie stood at the front of an auditorium the size of Utah, on Earth. She hadn't sought the position she was in, but also didn't feel like she could resist taking it. Her actions had led to this, how could she fail to follow through?

As she spoke, she leaned over and manipulated her Pyxis, which was blown up in size behind her so that everyone, no matter how far away, could see it. She looked at the image of Dominick, moving around the garage, preparing, once again, to end his life.

"This is an art, not a science. This is about knowing the people you watch over, and how the different paths of their lives will play out. We can't just pay attention to what they want at any given moment, because humans are so imperfect, what they want will often lead them to more unhappiness. We need to learn to read their hearts, their true selves, their souls. A person's soul never desires the wrong thing. It is incapable of that. A person's soul only wants to connect, to feel, to belong."

She waved her hand at the image behind her. Dominick was lying down in his truck, preparing to die. "This young man is preparing to commit suicide. So. Is that good, or is that bad? Is it harmful to him, or does it help him accomplish what his soul cries out for?"

She looked up at the faces of the millions who stared at her, rapt.

"There are no absolutes. Will you make mistakes? Yes. That is part of our learning process here, just as it is for those still on Earth. In this case, I have watched over this soul for three lifetimes. I know that with this person, his heart, his mind, and his soul, are all in alignment. The right thing for me to do here is to watch. And to feed the Machine with his pain and despair."

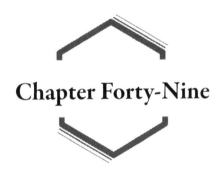

Chapter Forty-Nine

This time, Dominick opened his eyes, knowing exactly what to expect. Sure enough, Connie was sitting on his chest, looking worried. He sat up, hugged her, and said, "It's okay, Squig. I'm okay."

Relieved, she smiled and said, "Bubby's burning."

"Yeah, I know, I'm sitting on lava. Game's over for right now. C'mon, help me pick up the cushions, but be careful not to knock the lamp over and break it."

The extraordinary had become, if not commonplace, at least accepted.

Second time I died, I had no idea if I would even wake up again, and if so, where would I be. This time, I'm starting to figure it out.

Dominick looked down at his hands, small and childish once again, where they had been lean and strong, just a few moments before.

Now, I've got the prison stretch of childhood ahead of me. I'll bet people would think it would be great to be a kid again, no bills or responsibilities, but they haven't had to live the reality. People don't listen to you when you're a kid, no matter what you have to say. Your life is constantly under the control of someone else. It sucks.

An image of Emily crossed his mind and a small smile crossed his face.

But you're worth it, Em.

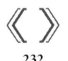

THE DEATH AND LIFE OF DOMINICK DAVIDNER

DESPITE HIS RESERVATIONS, Dominick slipped easily back into being a nine year old again
Fourth time's the charm.

He did his best to make small improvements in both his life and the people he loved as he lived through well-trod ground. He had learned that his father was willing to listen to him about using chewing tobacco, so he made sure to have that conversation with him each life. Dominick dreamed about having both his parents there the day he and Emily got married.

The years passed no more quickly the fourth time through than they had the two previous. He still spent too much time bored, casting about for things to keep himself occupied. He still started the small engine repair business, but this time he took a longer view of his future, as well. He planned accordingly, doing his best to use his scant knowledge of the future financial markets to make his plans.

More than anything, he wondered and worried about Emily.
Is she okay? Is she even alive? How do I know?

Dominick still had her number in Sheboygan memorized, and he put it to use. Every year, from the time he was once again fifteen years old, Dominick snuck away to the same payphone. He stacked the quarters on the steel shelf and dialed her number. The operator answered, told him how much the first three minutes would be, and then connected him.

He made the call each year on what had been their anniversary. The phone would brrrrrr in his ear and someone would answer. Most years, it was Louise Esterhaus, but on rare occasions, Harvey would answer. As time passed, Emily herself would often answer.

When she did, Dominick said a silent prayer of thanks, knowing that she would be alive in his mind, at least, for another year, then would quickly hang up. When Louise or Harvey answered, Dominick would say, "Can I speak to Emily, please?" then hold his breath, the memory of the phone call from his previous life still on his mind. Year after year, he got responses that varied from, "Can I tell her who's calling, please?" to a gruff, "She's not here," from Harvey. As soon as he knew she was alive still, he would hang up.

After he had made his annual call in 1977, he hung up, knees weak with relief that Emily herself had answered the phone. *One of these days, Caller ID will be invented, and they'll be able to see that these strange calls come from Emeryville, California. When did Caller ID become popular, anyway? Sometime in the eighties, right? I should have paid better attention to all these little details in my first life.*

Dominick graduated from high school again in 1977, once again with a sterling, if not-quite-perfect GPA. He once again took part in enough activities to get accepted at Cabrillo College. One blessing for him was that he hadn't actually made it to college in his two previous lives, so when the fall semester started, he was glad to have a semi-new experience to live through.

Once he got to college, he realized that he had been suffering a low-grade depression the previous nine years. Being shot, then recycled time and again can have that effect on you. But he bloomed a bit when college started, glad to have a new challenge.

From his perspective, it had been almost twenty years since he had seen Emily, and she felt further away than she ever had. He still made his annual call to her parent's house in Sheboygan, but now he was told, "She's away at college, can I take a message?"

He did his best to think of Emily as little as possible, but she was never far from his mind. Over the years, doubts began to set in.

What if I go through all this, and she's married by the time I catch up to her in this life? I can't do this again, I just can't.

Or, *If we are what I have always believed we are, soul mates, would she have really rejected me the way she did? Wouldn't we have found a way to work through it?*

In the end, he did the only thing he could—he lived his life day by day, just like every other soul on planet Earth.

Dominick finished his four year degree at Cabrillo College, which had turned out to be the perfect spot for him to go to school. Because he was a California resident, his tuition was low, and much of it was covered by scholarships. It was close enough that he could go home and check on his family when he wanted, but not so close that it needed to be every weekend, or even every month.

His folks had sold the little house in Emeryville just after he graduated with his teaching degree, because they couldn't believe how much it fetched on the open market. He wanted to tell them to hold on to it a few years longer, but decided not to interfere that much in their lives.

Once he had his degree, Dominick knew he wasn't ready to start teaching again just yet. He was twenty-two years old, he was finally in a part of his life that he hadn't lived over and over, and he didn't feel like walking down the same road he had in his first life.

So, he went adventuring.

Chapter Fifty

In his second life, Dominick told his parents he was going on a drive to see what he could see, but then had beelined straight for Sheboygan. In his fourth life, he really did go on a walkabout. After he graduated in June 1981, he drove south, to the beaches of Southern California.

He gave being a surfer his best shot. In the end, though, he found that surfing was another sport that he was not naturally talented at. He drank a few gallons of seawater, then figured his time was better spent getting a tan on solid ground. He did manage to find a job working in a surf shop, and the owner, not to mention most of the girls who came into the shop, took a shine to him. The shop owner, Ted, let him stay in a tiny room above the shop.

For a year, that was enough for him, and he was happy.

Then, a man named Craig Simmons started hanging around the store. Craig was taking a few months off, living the good life, preparing for a season spent as a smokejumper in Arizona.

That sounded exotic and interesting to Dominick, so he asked questions. What he got in return, was stories. Stories that involved risk, danger, and excitement. Dominick was hooked. It was too late for him to join up with Craig that year. You don't just walk in one day and become a smokejumper the next. Dominick had never flown, let alone jumped out of an airplane. He had no idea how to combat a wildfire in a remote area.

He knew he could learn, though, and so he gave his notice at the surf shop and drove to Missoula, Montana, where he learned to be a smokejumper. He also learned that although he had been sure he was in good shape, he had been horribly wrong. After he finished smokejumper school, *then* he was in good shape. Able to jump out of a plane, haul a 110-pound pack over miles of rough terrain, then wake up the next morning and do it again.

The following season, he caught on with the National Forest Service's West Yellowstone Smokejumpers. During fire season, Dominick stayed so busy traveling from one hot spot in the western United States to another, he was able to forget about his situation, about missing Emily. Then, the season passed, and he would be assigned to a ranger station in some remote area, and he had too much time to think.

After two years of that, he knew the hard work was great, but the downtime was too much, so he got in his truck and drove south again. He didn't stop until he saw the bright lights of the Las Vegas Strip. He wasn't a gambler, but he loved the excitement of The Strip, especially after the long hours of quiet contemplation high atop observation stations.

He had enough money saved from his Forest Service job that he didn't need to find work immediately, but it was April 1985, and Dominick was sure he remembered that Microsoft stock would be available soon. He wanted to buy as many shares as he could, just to ensure that he, and hopefully, Emily, would not have to worry about money in the future, despite whatever modest salaries they might have as teachers.

He couldn't remember exactly what year the Microsoft stock debuted, but he had been able to do enough research to find out that the company existed, and was growing rapidly. As soon as he got to Las Vegas, he found an investment advisor named Tom Patterson in the phone book and made an appointment for the next day.

When Dominick arrived the following morning, the receptionist looked him over, from his long, curly hair, to his work shirt, jeans and boots. She welcomed him and sat him in the outer office, then disappeared. A moment later, she was back, and said, "I'm sorry, but Mr. Patterson has been called away unexpectedly. Ms. Jansen will be right with you, though."

Dominick smiled to himself. *I guess I don't look like Howard Hughes, dressed this way, so they've shuffled me off to a junior associate. Whatever. I don't really need investing advice. Just someone to buy the shares for me when they come available.*

Ten minutes later, a tall, gray-haired woman with her hair pulled back into a bun, came around the corner. "Hello, Mr. ..."

"Davidner," Dominick said.

"Yes, Davidner. Very good. Please, come with me."

On the way to her tiny office, they passed an expansive office with a huge window that opened toward the Strip. A man sat with his cowboy boots on the desk, leaned back in his chair.

I would be willing to bet that is the absent Mr. Patterson.

When they reached Ms. Jansen's office, she said, "So, what can I do for you, Mr. Davidner?"

"Has Microsoft made their IPO yet?"

"Microsoft? Oh, no. They haven't even set a date for that. Why?"

"I want to buy at least a few hundred shares when it comes available. I know you can't tell me for sure, but what would you guess the shares will open at?"

"Mr. Davidner, this is Las Vegas. If you wish to gamble, there are many easier ways to do so than to go through this firm."

"Please. Humor me."

"There's no way to be sure, of course, but I might guess, maybe $15.00 per share."

Dominick did some quick math, taking that number and how much he had saved over the previous few years. *Might have to get a second job.*

"I just got into town, so I don't have an address or phone number, but I will soon. Can I get a card from you, so we can stay in touch?"

"Of course," she said, handing Dominick a card from her drawer. "But, really, I have to advise you against putting all your liquid assets into a new stock like that. They are often highly volatile, and many times, they crash. I would recommend a less-risky portfolio, filled with blue chip stocks, like IBM or General Motors. I know it's tempting at your age to look for a big win, but you have so many investing years ahead of you, boring is beautiful."

"Thank you. I'll take that under advisement. I appreciate you meeting with me.

Chapter Fifty-One

Dominick found a run-down apartment just off the northern end of The Strip that had affordable rents. He later learned that the place was cheap because a B-movie star had hanged himself in his unit two years before, and everyone believed it to be haunted.

Fine with me. I don't mind one more ghost, but I would guess he is probably laboring away at some earlier part of his life at this very moment, and not hanging around here watching me.

Las Vegas in 1985 was not as glitzy and glamorous as it would become in another ten years. The mega-resorts with faux Eiffel Towers, exploding volcanos and sinking pirate ships were not even a dream yet.

Dominick put his application in up and down The Strip and Downtown Vegas. The first interview he got was to be a bartender at a small bar in The Sands. The woman who conducted the interview thought Dominick would present the perfect image for the casino—as long as he was willing to get a haircut, which he was.

He worked five nights a week at the Silver Queen Lounge. The pay wasn't much, but his tips were good. Meanwhile, he attended school once again, spending his days learning how to be a blackjack dealer.

Within a month, he had graduated and got a job dealing downtown, at Binion's. Between working two full-time jobs on opposite ends of The Strip, he didn't have time to think too much, and definitely didn't have time to spend what he was earning.

During the five years since he had graduated from college, Dominick continued to call Emily once a year, on what had been their anniversary. Her parents were no longer as forthcoming with information about her, but Dominick could tell by their responses that she was still alive, if nothing else.

She might be married, with 2.5 kids, but at least she's alive.

All the double shifts were worth it to him. On January 3rd, he got a call from Ms. Jansen telling him that the Microsoft IPO was scheduled for March. Dominick checked his bank balance. Between what he had saved on Forest Service duty and working himself into the ground since he had arrived in Vegas, he had $6,200 stashed away. He thought that even if the IPO opened higher than what Ms. Jansen it would, he still might have enough to buy 200 shares.

I sure wish I had paid more attention to this stuff the first time around. I remember that Microsoft stock split a bunch of times, and went up a lot, but I have idea what that means in practical dollars and sense. Does 200 original shares give me drop dead money for the rest of my life, or just enough to be better off than most other teachers? I guess I'll buy it, forget it, and find out in another ten years or so.

When March 13 rolled around, Ms. Jansen, against her wishes, invested the entire $6,000 he gave her into Microsoft stock at 24.12 per share. Not quite as good as the $21.00 it opened at, but Dominick didn't care. He felt like he had one more thing he could tick off his *Lifetime #4 To-Do List*.

He had come to like the financial cushion he had built up over the previous few years, and now that it was invested, he decided to continue working the double shifts at The Sands and Binion's until he had a decent amount built back up. Dominick lived frugally, though, and after another three months of working both jobs, he felt like he could give one of them up. He kept the job working at the Sands, because he was a night owl, and that suited his normal circadian rhythm.

After working close to eighty hours a week for the previous eighteen months, cutting back to one job felt like a vacation. The relief of that soon passed, though, and he was once again bored and restless. The job bartending at The Sands was repetitive. New tourists came in every night, but they all looked alike after seeing so many of them.

He checked his bank balance, found it healthy again, and put his notice in. He did the same at the tiny apartment he had rented, and was once again unfettered.

Dominick celebrated his 27th birthday on his last day in Las Vegas. He had lived there eighteen months, but aside from work acquaintances, he hadn't made any close friends. Being a multi-life time traveler had its drawbacks, and one of them was that he felt removed from most people, separate.

He felt the need to connect with someone, though, so he called home.

Connie had graduated from high school several years before, and had decided to go to work instead of going to school. Sam was a fully licensed electrician, and had finally moved out and gotten his own place. Laura and Joe were in their early fifties now. They had moved from Emeryville, north to Middle Falls, Oregon, which had caught Dominick off-guard initially. He'd had nothing to do with their decision to move, which had been predicated on Joe getting a supervisory role in a new job, and that got him off his feet at least part of the day. He hadn't visited them since they had moved earlier that year. Even with Joe's new job, they were both still working too hard, at least in Dominick's opinion. .

He found a payphone and dialed their number. *Maybe if this stock really takes off, I can help them out. Pay off their mortgage or something, so they can take it easier.*

Laura answered the phone. "Hello?"

"Hey, Mom. What's up?"

"What's up with you, Mr. Birthday Boy?! Your dad just asked if we had heard from you yet. How is life in the desert?"

"It's a little boring, Mom. I'm going to move on again, do something else. Would it be okay if I drove up there and spent a few days with you guys while I decide what's next?"

"Oh, Nicky, you know you never need to ask. It's been way too long since we've seen you!" Over her shoulder, she shouted, "Joe, Nicky's coming home!"

Faintly, in the distance, he heard the familiar voice say, "About damn time. I thought he'd disowned us." Closer, he heard Joe say, "Come home, Nicky. We miss you."

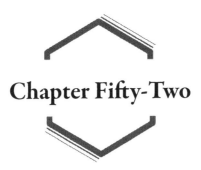

Chapter Fifty-Two

Dominick pulled into his parent's new home, on the outskirts of Middle Falls, Oregon, after midnight the following day. He'd called ahead and let them know he would be getting in late, so they left the front door unlocked for him.

Inside the neat little one story house, Dominick found a bed made up for him on the couch. Joe and Laura had a spare bedroom, but they hadn't set it up for company since they had moved. There was a fluffy pillow at one end of the couch, with a note in his mother's elegant handwriting: "Welcome home, Nicky."

After driving straight through the day before, Dominick fell asleep immediately and slept straight through until after 10:00 am the next morning. He woke up to find another note on the coffee table.

"See you tonight. I'll make dinner. Mom."

Either they were very quiet this morning while they were getting ready for work, or I was dead to the world.

Dominick spent the day rattling around the empty house, trying to find things that would keep him busy and help his parents at the same time. He didn't feel he could do any of the remaining unpacking for them, but he was able to mow the lawn, and he fixed a loose gutter on the side of the house.

He even surprised Laura by having dinner ready for her when she came home. He had taught himself to cook during his bachelor years, and he made a very passable spaghetti.

"What's that I smell?" Laura asked as soon as she opened the door.

"You've worked hard all day, Mom," Dominick said, wrapping her in a long hug. "You don't have to cook, too. Men are not helpless, you know."

She laughed, and said, "Have you met your brother? As much as he loves his food, you'd think he'd learn how to cook but he and the kitchen go together like a garbage disposal and a spoon." She reached up to hold his face in both hands. "Don't stay gone so long, Nicky."

The door opened and Joe strode through. He grabbed Dominick around the neck and hugged him too. "You're twenty-seven years old. When are you going to stop growing?"

"Six foot tall, Dad, just like I have been for ten years. I think you might just be shrinking."

"Still big enough to take you down a peg or two."

Dominick hugged him back. It was like hugging corded steel. *I believe you could, Dad.*

Over dinner, Dominick told them what it was like living in Las Vegas, *The City That Never Sleeps*.

Laura had just one question. "Did you meet any nice girls?"

Dominick held up his hands in a weighing motion. "Nice girls," he said lowering his left hand, "Las Vegas," and he lowered his right. "Showgirls? Yes, plenty. Cocktail waitresses? By the dozen." For a moment, he flashed back on announcing that Sam had called Billy Stitts' sister a whore, and how upset Laura had been at the use of that word in her house. *Guess I'll leave them off the list.* "But, nice girls, the kind you bring home to Mom and Dad? Nope, not a one."

Laura sighed. "Looks like I'm going to have to rely on Connie to give me grandbabies to spoil, since you and your brother are such late starters."

Let's see, 1987. That's right. This is the year that Connie will meet Jim. They'll get married next year, and she'll finally give Mom those grandchildren the year after that.

"Has Connie met anyone?" Dominick asked innocently.

"As a matter of fact, she has."

"What's his name?" *I know the answer, but I'll play along.*

"Charlie. Charlie Meeks. We haven't met him yet, but he's a dentist in the same clinic where she works."

Dominick had already been nodding in agreement, but stopped abruptly. "Wait. What? Charlie? Not Jim?"

"Jim?" Laura said, puzzlement written across her furrowed brow.

Dominick shook his head. "Never mind. I just heard you wrong."

Laura went on, telling Dominick all about this Charlie, and how well he and Connie got on. Dominick didn't hear any of it.

Charlie? I know things are different each life. Different things happen. But I've spent eighteen years in this life for one reason—hoping Emily will be here at the right time. That we are fated to be together. But, Connie and Jim were great together too. They loved each other. And now, she's with the wrong guy. Maybe he's the right guy for this life but he's not Jim.

"Did you hear what I said, honey?" Laura said, snapping Dominick out of his reverie.

"Huh? Oh, sure Mom. He sounds like a great guy. I'm sure they'll be cranking up the baby factory for you any day now."

"Oh, pshh. Stop it now." She plucked a piece of garlic bread and wound a bite of spaghetti on her fork. "So, what's next? You've got a good four year degree wasting away, and you're gallivanting around the country playing firefighter and bartender. When are you going to get some use out of that diploma?"

It's like she's playing all of Mom's Greatest Hits. I guess it really has been too long between visits, so she's got all her little nags lined up.

"Actually, Mom, I've been thinking about settling down and doing some teaching."

"Well, praise the Lord!" Laura cupped her hands together and glanced to the heavens. That makes me so happy, Nicky." She reached over and squeezed his hand. A thought occurred to her. "Oh! I heard from Janet at work that they were looking for a teacher at the high school here in town."

"Really? It's August. They should have all their staff in place." *I was hoping to maybe sub this year and catch on next year.*

"They did, but Mr. Carmichael just recently became ill, and he's not going to teach this year."

I don't ever remember meeting a Carmichael at Middle Falls High. Interesting.

"I'm sure they'll be looking for someone soon, though. School starts in just a few weeks. Maybe you should go down and apply in person."

"Sure, Mom. I sure will."

"Oh, Nicky. It would be so wonderful to have you working here. It's really a nice little town."

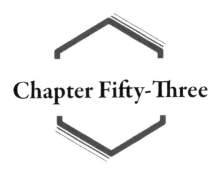

Chapter Fifty-Three

The next morning, Dominick got up early, showered, and was dressed in his best "teacherly" outfit—khaki slacks and a blue button down shirt—by 8:30 am. He grabbed a quick cup of his mom's coffee and jumped in his truck.

Driving into town, on the familiar roads to the high school, he had an intense feeling of déjà vu.

Keep it together. It's been an eighteen year journey to get here, but I'm still freaked out that Connie is getting serious with the wrong guy. If I've lived all this time just to get this shot, then I find out it was all for nothing, I don't know what I'll do. I can't do this again. I think I'll go crazy if I try.

He parked in the employee parking lot of Middle Falls High. It was still August, and school was out, but Dominick knew that at least some of the staff would be there, getting things ready for the new school year.

He went directly to the office and recognized Sandra Mullins immediately. She had been sitting behind the desk of that office, keeping any number of different principles organized for decades. She had still been sitting there the last time Dominick had seen her, in his first life.

Glad to see some things haven't changed.

"Hello," Dominick said, as though he didn't know her. "My name is Dominick Davidner. I'm a teacher, looking for a job."

Mrs. Mullins looked him up and down, then said, "How fortuitous. Let me get Mr. James for you."

That threw Dominick for another loop. *There was no Mr. James who acted as principal, or anything, when I was at Middle Falls. So many changes popping up. Likely, I would have noticed them before now, but I was off breaking a new trail, so I didn't.*

Mrs. Mullins came back from the inner office, accompanied by a short, heavy-set man. He was balding, but with a fringe of copper hair.

"Mr. Davidner, Mrs. Mullins tells me that you are a teacher. We've had a bit of an unplanned occurrence this week, so I'm happy to see you. Please come in."

Once inside his office, Mr. James said, "Do you have a resume with you?"

Dominick shook his head and said, "No, sir. I'm afraid this is a little spur of the moment. Until just a few days ago, I was living in Las Vegas. I came up to visit with my parents, and at dinner last night, my mom mentioned that you might be looking for someone."

"And, were you teaching in Las Vegas?"

"Well, no." Anticipating the next question, Dominick said, "I was a bartender there. Oh, and a blackjack dealer."

"But," Mr. James said, searching for something, anything, "you have taught before?"

It's been a few lifetimes ago, but sure I have. I could walk you to my classroom right now.

"No, sir."

Mr. James winced. "I see. So, no resume, no experience. You do have a degree, don't you?"

"Yes, sir. Cabrillo College in Santa Cruz."

"Good! Well, that's something." He glanced at the calendar on his desk. "School starts three weeks from Monday. Our regular English teacher, Mr. Carmichael, has taken a rather sudden leave of absence. How are you with the subject?"

"It's what I love most."

"Who's your favorite author?"

"Vonnegut, but I love to teach Dickens."

"Very good."

Tough interviewer. I needed to know the names of two authors.

"Well, marry in haste, repent in leisure. I'm sure you understand. We're having a board meeting this evening to decide our path. I'll be in touch with you. Please, leave your number with Mrs. Mullins."

"Thank you. I appreciate the opportunity."

He pulled out of the high school parking lot and checked his watch. Only 10:15. Way too early to go home and sit around the house waiting for his parents to come home. Without realizing where he was going, he drove to Middle Falls Elementary, where Emily had taught.

She didn't start there until 1988 though. We met at a district teacher's meeting just before school that year. So, what's that, then, another year? After all the waiting I've been doing, I can do that standing on my head.

He drove past the school and pulled into the parking lot to turn around and head back toward downtown. *Maybe see what's playing at the Pickwick. Did they have matinees during the week?*

Then, Dominick's mind went blank. Coming out the back doors of the school were two women, both carrying stacks of books. One was an older woman, with gray hair and glasses. The other was Emily.

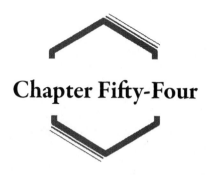

Chapter Fifty-Four

Emily. You're here now?

He stopped the truck and jumped out. He jogged up to the two women.

"Can we help you?" the older woman asked.

"Actually, I was thinking I could help you. I thought maybe I could carry those books for you."

"Well, thank you," the older woman said. "Are you a knight in shining armor, wandering the countryside, looking for good deeds to perform?"

Think fast.

"Actually, I just interviewed with Mr. James over at the high school for the English teacher's position. I thought I'd drive around town and check out what the rest of the district looks like."

He risked one glance at Emily. Her hair was shorter than when he had last seen her in Sheboygan. She was so lovely she stunned him into silence.

Thank you, God.

He did his best to recover his senses. "I'm Dominick Davidner. I'm new in town. My parents just moved here, and when I came to visit them, they told me about the job at the high school."

The older woman handed her stack of books to Dominick. "I'm Mrs. Bilas, Mr. Davidner. And I will never look a gift horse in the mouth. We're carrying these back to the storage room in this building."

Dominick balanced her stack of books in his arms, then reached out, offering to take Emily's as well. "Mrs...?"

"Miss," Emily said with a dazzling smile that warmed Dominick all the way down to his cowboy boots. "Emily Esterhaus."

Thank you...Thank you, thank you, thank you.

"Pleased to meet you, Mrs. Bilas, and Miss Esterhaus."

The women led Dominick along the sidewalk and into a storage room. They indicated an empty spot on a shelf in the back and Dominick stacked the books neatly there. He dusted his hands against his khakis and said, "Is that it? Any more?"

The two women looked at each other and laughed. Mrs. Bilas said, "Are you looking for a full time job today? We've got a few hundred books we still need to move. We had just been talking about seeing if the kindergarten class had a wagon we could borrow."

"Until my folks get home from work tonight, I am completely available. Feel free to use and abuse me."

"Well, Emily, if you've got this strapping young man to help you, I think I can go back to my own classroom."

Thank you, Mrs. Bilas. I think I love you.

"Show me the way, ma'am," Dominick said to Emily.

"I am thankful for your help, but if you call me 'ma'am' again, all bets are off." She stopped and squinted at Dominick. "I'd be willing to bet you are *quite* a bit older than me."

Dominick pointed at his chest and said, "27."

Emily nodded. "I knew it. I am only 26."

"Yes, that is a substantial difference," Dominick said.

Emily. It's like we have never been apart. I love you!

The two of them spent the next ninety minutes hauling dozens of copies of *The World of Science* and *Primary Mathematics* textbooks to the storage room, then unboxing new textbooks. Dominick had a difficult time keeping the smile from his face, but did his best. He didn't want Emily to think he was mentally challenged.

When the last of the books were unboxed, Emily said, "I think I owe you something for all this. Will you settle for a burger and fries at the Burger Pit?"

I haven't heard that name in three decades. Will I settle for the most delicious hamburger in three states with the most beautiful girl around who just happens to be the one true love of my life? You know it.

"The Burger Pit, huh? Sounds like my kind of place. I'll go, but we've got to split the tab, okay? If my mom hears that I let the first beautiful girl I meet pay for my meal, she'd skin me alive."

They rode to the Burger Pit in Emily's yellow Chevette.

Man, these Chevettes. They're small, but they make up for it by being slow. If you're gonna drive one of these, you need a mechanic in the family.

At lunch, they made small talk about Middle Falls. Emily told Dominick that she was new in town, too, that she had just arrived from Wisconsin to take this job teaching third grade. Dominick told her a little about being a fire jumper and working in the casinos in Las Vegas. He managed to get through the whole lunch without blurting out that he loved her. He considered that a moral victory.

Lunch was finished much too soon for Dominick's tastes. Before he knew it, they had thrown their trash away, and Emily had driven back to the school. She pulled around to the back parking lot and stopped by Dominick's *Ugly Truckling*.

"Thank you for all the help. I would have been at it all day. And, good luck with your job interview. I hope you get it."

"Me too," Dominick said with a broad grin.

Damn. What do I do? Ask her out? Ask for her phone number? Don't want to be too forward.

Dominick climbed out of the Chevette, then leaned down to say goodbye. When he did, he saw that Emily was jotting something down on a slip of paper. "Here," she said. "This is my number. You can call me sometime, if you want."

"Sure will," Dominick said, because those were the only two words in his head.

Dominick got in his truck and floated home.

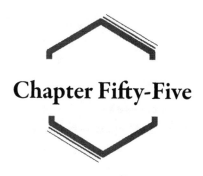

Chapter Fifty-Five

At dinner that night. Dominick told his parents, "I met a girl today."

This was met with more excitement than when he had told them how his job interview had gone, at least by Laura. Joe mostly smiled to himself and kept eating.

"Well, you can't just say something like that and then leave it lying there. I need details!"

"After my interview, I was just driving around town, checking things out. I turned around in the parking lot of the elementary school, and saw two ladies carrying heavy books, so I jumped out to help them."

"I always raised you to be a gentleman."

"One of them, her name is Emily, needed more help, so I stuck around her classroom and helped her get things organized. Then, we went to lunch."

"Well, that's a good start."

Dominick nodded. "I'm going to marry her."

That got even Joe's attention. He put down his fork, took a pull on his Budweiser and looked long and hard at Dominick. "You're twenty-seven years old, and never even had a serious girlfriend, unless you've been hiding her, so you might want to slow down a bit. Go on a few dates. You've always been too impetuous. Marriage is nothing to take lightly. Not all pretty girls running around out there are as perfect as your mother is."

"But, Dad. How many times did you need to meet Mom before you knew you were going to get married."

"Once."

"What?" Laura said. This was obviously news to her.

"I saw you at that dance. You were with that Falkner boy. I knew he wasn't right for you. And I knew I was."

"The things you learn after 35 years of marriage," Laura said. Her eyes twinkled at the memory.

"So, doesn't that prove my point, then, Dad?"

"In a way, but I didn't go around telling everyone I was going to marry your Mom, just because I knew it. Some things are better kept under your hat. You don't want to scare 'em off too early. Women are mysterious, divine creatures. Men, well, we're not. So we've got to sneak up on 'em a little bit."

Dad, the dating philosopher. Who knew?

OVER THE NEXT FEW MONTHS, Dominick did his best to "sneak up on her a little bit." He got the job teaching English at Middle Falls High, and he saw Emily every chance he got, but not *too* often.

The last time I saw Emily, everything seemed so much harder. I had to pursue her. Every step I took was like walking in wet cement. Everything I did pushed her further away.

An image flashed through his mind: his father, back in their little one car garage, putting the tools away after working on a project. "A place for everything, Nicky, and everything in its place." *And, a time for everything, and everything in its time. I wonder why it took me four lifetimes to figure that out. No matter whether something is meant to be or not, it won't happen until its own time.*

Dominick had moved off his parents' couch as soon as he had gotten the job teaching English at Middle Falls High. He still had dinner with them a few times a week, but it was important to set up his own life, too.

After they had been dating for a month, Dominick bowed to parental pressure and brought Emily home for dinner. He watched with a little wonder as his father met Emily. Joe reached out to shake her hand, but she would have none of that. She wrapped him in a hug that surprised him so much that Dominick laughed a little.

You never had the chance to meet her, Dad. It means a lot that you can, now.

Around the dinner table, Laura quizzed Emily—about her family, what college had been like, what Wisconsin was like, and, finally, whether she wanted to have children.

Dominick tried to throw himself in front of the speeding train of questions, but Emily reached out and laid her hand on his. "It's okay. Really. I'd love to have children."

Laura smiled at her, and Dominick could see Emily had her blessing. He never doubted how his dad felt. From the first hug on, he could see that Joe felt the same that Dominick himself did.

The following summer, Dominick took a job with a roofing company, just to bring in a little extra money. He followed his Microsoft stock in the newspaper occasionally, but it hadn't really started to take off yet.

Things change from life to life. Maybe a totally different company will take off in this world. Doesn't matter too much one way or the other.

He worked long hours putting roofs on houses that summer, because he wanted to buy a ring. He wanted something nicer than he had bought that fateful second time he had asked Emily to marry him, but he didn't want to cash in any of his shares yet. He had other plans for that money, if and when it arrived.

So he hammered nails in the sun, got a great tan, and stayed in shape that summer. He also squirreled away an extra couple of thousand dollars.

On the one year anniversary of the day he had helped Emily stack books, he asked her to go to Portland with him, and to pack a bag.

He made reservations at the Sentinel Hotel, and for dinner at the El Gaucho. Not coincidentally, these were the same places he'd had reservations on their tenth anniversary, which was thirty-seven years ago, from Dominick's perspective.

They checked into the historic hotel in early afternoon and got dressed in their best—Dominick in his one suit, Emily in a black cocktail dress that made Dominick wish it was something she wore more often.

Even though they were in their late twenties, and Dominick was much older than that every way but physically, they still felt like little kids playing dress up as they walked through the doors of the El Gaucho. The interior of the restaurant was dimly lit, but the whole atmosphere, from the leather booths, to the deep pile carpeting, to the open beam ceiling, linen tablecloths, and candle light, made them feel like they were part of a fairy tale.

"Nicky!" Emily whispered in his ear. "This place must be so expensive!"

"Why do you think I've been working all summer?"

"I can't believe you worked so hard just so we could come blow it in one night!"

"You're worth it."

They were seated halfway to the back of the restaurant, at a table up on a slight riser, so they were able to look out at all the other diners.

"I'm not sure I know which fork to use for what!" Emily said, looking at the array of cutlery spread out in front of her.

"Just don't use your knife to eat your soup, or your spoon to cut your steak, and you'll be fine."

Dominick ordered for both of them, because he knew Emily would order whatever was least expensive on the menu.

Not tonight, Em. Tonight, we splurge.

After they worked their way through the crab cocktail appetizer, clam chowder, and filet mignon, Dominick ordered Bananas Foster for them.

"I'm not actually sure what Bananas Foster is, but I guess we'll find out!"

To the surprise of both of them, it turned out to be not only delicious, but also cooked right at their table, including a flaming finish.

Dominick had been nervous all evening, not because of their surroundings, but because of the small black box he carried in his suit pocket. His mind wandered back to the last, disastrous time he had done this, but he pushed those thoughts away.

Emily nudged her dessert plate away with half her Bananas Foster left and said, "I will never eat again. Are you trying to fatten me up?"

Dominick didn't answer. His mouth felt too dry to speak. He slipped out of his side of the booth and realized that because they were sitting on a riser, there was no place to kneel. He shrugged, stood close to Emily, and produced the box.

Emily's eyes grew wide. She said, "Oh." Her hands went to her mouth.

This is where everything went sideways last time. Please, God. If you can answer one prayer for me in this string of mixed up lives, let it be this one. Let her say 'yes.'

"Emily Esterhaus, I know we've only known each other for a year, but I can't imagine ever finding someone as perfect as you are. Will you marry me?"

Tears spilled out of Emily's eyes. She smiled and reached for Dominick. Her hands were shaking. "Yes."

It was all she needed to say. Dominick's head dropped, and he said a silent prayer of thanks.

Dominick leaned toward her and kissed her, softly at first, then like he meant it. When their lips parted, he realized that they were both crying.

The tables around them had turned to watch the drama play out. A man at the booth next to them said, "Well, what did she say?"

Dominick flashed a thumbs-up to him, and all the tables around them burst into applause.

He leaned in close to Emily and whispered in her ear, "I guess even rich people appreciate a good love story."

Chapter Fifty-Six

After much back and forth, they decided to get married the next summer, after school was out. Emily wanted to give her parents and friends from Wisconsin enough warning so they could travel for the wedding. Dominick briefly lobbied for a date in December—their original wedding date—but changed his mind and let Emily pick the date. She wanted to be a June bride, and who was he to stand in her way?

A time for everything and everything in its time.

They were new to Middle Falls so they planned a small wedding. Still, Emily managed to talk her two best friends from college—Sandy and Melody—to fly out and be her co-Maids of Honor. Dominick was proud to ask Joe to stand up with him as his Best Man, and Sam to be his only groomsman. Sam had grown up in the years Dominick had been away. He had a good job, and he even brought a girl to the wedding, giving Laura dreams of being a grandmother on three fronts.

It was that odd sense of déjà vu that Dominick never got used to when he met Melody and Sandy for the first time in this lifetime. They were exactly the same, just a little older. The first thing Melody said was, "Oh, he's a cute one. Are all the Oregon boys this cute? I might have to move out here!"

They held the wedding at Middle Falls park, right next to the actual falls, which weren't spectacular, but were nonetheless the town's namesake. The wedding was small. Including Connie and her new fiancée, Charlie, Sam and Belinda, his new girlfriend, Harvey and Louise Esterhaus, and all the Middle Falls teaching friends, there were still less than fifty people in attendance.

None of that mattered at all to Dominick. To him, he and Emily could have eloped to Reno, or gotten married at the local Justice of the Peace. After so many years and lifetimes of waiting, he just wanted it to happen.

Emily was highly spiritual, but not religious, so having the priest from the local Catholic Church perform the wedding was impossible. Instead, they asked their friend, Glenn Mobrey, the History teacher at Middle Falls High, who was also licensed to perform weddings, to do the honors.

Dominick, Joe, and Sam wore charcoal gray tuxedos. Emily's bridesmaids wore sunshine-yellow dresses that would undoubtedly hang in their closets unworn until they finally donated them to Goodwill in five or ten years. Emily wore a high-necked bridal gown and matching bridal hat. She was the very picture of a late-eighties bride.

At the appointed hour, Glenn Mobrey said, "I wrote a little speech today," and took a thick sheaf of papers out of his jacket pocket. The crowd groaned inwardly. "But it's a little hot out here, so I'm going to give you all a break and not deliver it." There were a few chuckles and a smattering of thankful applause.

"Seriously, though, I feel blessed to have the opportunity to help join these two shining spirits together in matrimony. Dominick did ask me to read a short verse, from Corinthians, so I will do that.

To everything there is a season, and a time to every purpose under the heaven:

A time to be born, and a time to die; a time to plant, and a time to pluck up that which is planted;

A time to kill, and a time to heal; a time to break down, and a time to build up.

"Today is definitely a day when we are joining together and building up. I have only known Dominick and Emily a short time, but they have both made an impression on me with their love and the way they have become such an important part of our local community. Dominick and Emily have written their own vows. Dominick?

Dominick took a deep breath, blew it out, and smiled nervously at his bride. "Emily, all my life, I knew something was missing. That day I saw you and Mrs. Bilas carrying those books across the parking lot, I found out what it was. I was missing someone who I could trust completely with all my life's secrets, knowing they would hold them deep in their heart and keep them safe. I was missing someone who I just had to tell about my day, all the good and the bad. I was missing someone to plan a future with, someone I could be myself with, and someone who would love me for who I am, all through my life. That very first day, I knew you were all these missing pieces and more. With you beside me, I never need to look backwards. Together, we can spend the rest of our lives looking forward. My vow to you is simple. I give you my life."

Behind Emily, Melody sniffed a little. Under her breath, she said, "Beautiful."

Emily wiped a tear away and said, "From the first moment I saw you, I knew we would always be together. You are my heart. I give you my life."

Mr. Mobrey smiled at both of them, and said, "Ladies and gentlemen, for the first time anywhere, may I present Mr. and Mrs. Dominick and Emily Davidner."

Dominick laughed. *Not exactly the first time anywhere, but I'll take it.*

He and Emily walked down the aisle, through all their friends and loved ones, and into the sunshine.

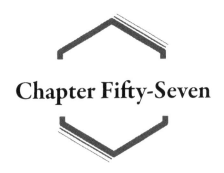

Chapter Fifty-Seven

The next ten years were not a carbon copy of their first life, and that was a relief for Dominick, too. Over the years, the stock he had bought in 1986 blossomed, and by 1996, his original 250 shares had blossomed into 4,500 shares, thanks to stock splits. At some point, Dominick realized he was a millionaire. It wasn't quite drop dead money, but he was certainly more comfortable than he would have been budgeting on two teacher's salaries.

He had told Emily about the Microsoft stock almost as an afterthought on their wedding day. She didn't believe him, but when he promised to put her on with his stock broker in Vegas the next day, she was convinced,

He was sure that the stock would continue to go up, at least until 1999, so he didn't want to divest or cash in too much of it, but he did sell enough shares that he was able to pay off his parent's mortgage, so Laura could stay home, and Joe could cut back his hours. He also cashed enough to put a down payment on a house. The rest they tucked away, hoping for more stock splits.

Life at the Davidner house was good, if not perfect. No marriage is perfect, even one as freighted with love and meaning as Dominick and Emily's. They still argued from time to time, and they were both disappointed at their ongoing inability to get pregnant. Both Sam and Connie had two children each, which eased the pressure from Laura and Joe, but not from Harvey and Louise, and not from themselves.

Still, their love never wavered, and they never said anything so horrible to each other that an apology couldn't heal it.

In 1998, Dominick celebrated his tenth anniversary teaching at Middle Falls Elementary. On the first day of that new school year, he welcomed his freshman English class. He looked up to see Gerald Fleischer sitting in the back row. Dominick flashed back to that day he had stormed his class with a gun in each hand and needed to sit down.

I guess I knew he would show up one of these days.

Dominick had been given decades to think about and worry what had happened at the end of his first life. Now, sitting twenty feet away from the boy who had murdered him, Dominick was still unsure.

What pushed him over the edge? Being bullied? Bad home life? Or, is he just a sociopath?

Dominick had no one he could talk about it with. He talked with Emily about everything else, but he had never found a way to tell her about his multiple lives. Maybe she would believe him, and it would be a relief to be able to talk with her about it. In the final analysis, he knew there was no way he could prove the truth, although he could give her a lot of circumstantial evidence. If he told her and she didn't believe him, where were they then? Very likely with a huge wedge between them. They were on much more solid ground than when he had blurted the truth out in Sheboygan two lives ago, but the downside was so much greater than the upside, that he held his own counsel. As his father had once told him, "Some things you just need to keep to yourself."

And now, here he was, face to face with his killer, and still no plan in place to deal with him.

He didn't bring the guns to school until December a year from now. I can't count on things happening the same way, but maybe I can make a change in his life.

At lunch that day, Dominick took his brown bag lunch to the teacher's lounge, just like he did every day. Emily had packed him some left over spaghetti and pasta salad. He popped the spaghetti into the microwave and sat down while it heated.

Zack Weaver was already sitting at the table, reading a book. Zack was a bright guy, but he wasn't a bookworm, so Dominick craned his head to see what he was reading. The title on the front showed the face of a frightened young boy. The title read, *The Unusual Second Life of Timothy Wallace*. The author's name at the bottom was Thomas Weaver.

"Relative of yours?"

"Yeah," Zack said. "My brother, actually. He's an attorney here in town, but in his spare time, he wrote this book, and he got it published." He took a bite of his sandwich and chewed it thoughtfully. "It's actually good. Who knew?"

"What's it about?"

"It's about this kid who accidentally kills his older, very good looking brother. I'm pretty sure he based that character on me."

"You'll never have self-confidence issues, Zack."

Ignoring him, Zack went on, "Killing his brother really messes him up, and he has a pretty terrible life, so he kills himself, then wakes up back in his teenage body, but he can remember everything that happened in his previous life."

The microwave beeped, but Dominick wasn't paying attention. "What?"

"I know, it sounds weird, but it's really pretty interesting. It's like he took our lives and threw them into a blender with a bunch of hallucinogenic drugs and this story came out."

"Hang on, hang on. Did you say he died, then woke up back in his own body and remembered his old life?"

"Mmm-hmmph" Zack said around a bite of peanut butter and jelly.

"Where can I get a copy?" Dominick asked, trying not to seem too eager.

Zack, engrossed in the book, didn't notice anything. "He's doing a signing at the bookstore in town tonight. Local writer makes good and all that, you know. It's kind of weird reading things that I remember happening and finding them in a book years later."

No, that's not weird. What's weird is, your brother has to be someone like me—someone living his life over again.

He pulled his spaghetti out of the microwave and slipped it back into the bag, then walked out of the lounge and into the sunshine. He grabbed his Nokia phone from the pocket of his khakis and pulled the antenna up. He held the 2 down a few seconds, and it dialed Emily.

"Hey, hon," she said. "Surviving the first day of school with your new set of monsters?"

Surviving. Yes, so far.

"So far, so good. Hey, I was just talking to Zack in the lounge. His brother wrote a book and he's signing it at the bookstore tonight at six. You wanna go?"

"That would be fun, but they've called a mandatory meeting for all of us."

"Nice thing to do on the first day."

"Yes, the new principal is not very popular at the moment."

"Okay, I think I'm gonna go. I want to read this book."

"K, hon. If I get home ahead of you, I'll heat up some of last night's leftovers."

"If I beat you there, I'll do the same. I love you, Em." That's the way he had said it to her every day since he had first told her. It was always "I love you," not "Love ya," or a rote "Love you, too." On the day he was killed, his last words to her were a smart aleck quip. This life, he made sure that wouldn't happen again—whenever their last goodbye was to be, she would have heard, "I love you, Emily," that day.

Dominick went back into the teacher's lounge and stashed his uneaten lunch back in the refrigerator and returned to class. He did his best to focus the rest of the day, but his mind swirled with the possibility of finally finding someone he could talk to.

Chapter Fifty-Eight

Dominick arrived at the bookstore, called *The Story Emporium*, at 5:30. There was a table set up at the front of the store, with a few rows of chairs. It didn't look like they were expecting a huge turnout. There were stacks of the hardback he had seen Zack reading on the table, but no one was around. Dominick plucked one off the top of the stack, then wandered the store, looking for something for Emily.

Gift giving had been easy for the first nine years of their marriage, because he still had memories of what she liked and didn't like. *Getting tougher, now. I am going to have to start getting creative again.*

He picked up *Bag of Bones,* Stephen King's new book, but put it back down. *That would be two for me and none for Emily. No good.*

He saw *Cold Mountain,* by Charles Frazier on a top shelf and pulled it down to read the back cover. *Hmm. A little history and romance combined. Ladies and Gentlemen, we've got a winner.*

He took both books up to the register and paid for them, then took up a seat in the back row of chairs at the front of the store. He cracked *The Unusual Second Life of Timothy Wallace* open.

The dedication page read, simply, "For Carrie."

The opening chapters of the book were set in 1976, and Dominick was immediately engrossed. He had lived through 1976 four times himself, and he remembered it well.

"You know, it makes new authors uneasy to see someone actually reading their book, right?"

Dominick jumped a little, then looked up to see a middle-aged man smiling down at him.

"Oh. Oh, is this yours?" Dominick asked, holding up the book.

"Sure is." The man held out his hand. "Thomas Weaver."

"Oh, hey. I'm Dominick. I'm actually a friend of your brother. We both teach at Middle Falls. I saw him reading it today and he mentioned you'd be here signing copies tonight, so I thought I'd swing by."

There. That's casual enough, right? I can't just blurt out, 'I'm a time traveler too!'

Dominick never would have pegged Thomas and Zack for brothers. Zack was tall and lean, with the kind of casual good looks that were destined to improve with age. Thomas was shorter, a few pounds overweight, and with a face that disappeared in a crowd.

I suppose most anyone comes off poorly if you compare them with Zack, though.

"I appreciate it. The girl at the register said the last local author they had in only had one person show up, so you make me at least equal with her. Take that, Edna."

"Zack said the book was a mixture of fact and fiction. It's about time travel, though, so I guess that's the fiction part, right?"

"There are more things in Heaven and Earth, Horatio, than are dreamt of in your philosophy."

"Dominick. My name's Dominick."

"Yeah, I know. That's Shakespeare. One of the horribly pretentious things authors do—quoting the Bard."

An elderly woman who had a large bag with her took another book off the stack on the table.

"You're doing land-office business, Thomas. I guess Edna can suck on your fumes."

Thomas looked at him, surprised, and laughed. He looked at his watch. "I've got to go get the little sign I had printed up. I'll be back in a minute."

While Thomas was gone, several other people sat down. By the time he got back, seven people were scattered around the seats. Thomas looked at Dominick with raised eyebrows. Dominick flashed him a thumbs up as though he was personally responsible for the new arrivals.

Thomas carried a rectangular sign with the cover of his book on it and set it up on an easel. He turned and smiled at the people in the crowd. He nodded at the bored girl behind the cash register.

She leaned over and clicked on a small microphone. "Local author Thomas Weaver is speaking at the front of the store, for anyone who is interested." Her tone of voice made it clear that she couldn't imagine anyone being interested.

"Okay, okay. Well, we'll just get started then. I'm going to do a little reading from my book, then I'll be happy to answer any questions for you. Please excuse me if I sound a little nervous. I'm a lot more comfortable addressing a judge and jury than I am doing this." He glanced up to see if that brought a chuckle from anyone, but saw only expectant faces.

He picked up a copy of his book and began to read.

Thomas read for about ten minutes. He read a part of the story where a fifty-three-year-old man killed himself, then woke up in his fifteen year old body.

Dominick was very interested.

After he read the last paragraph, Thomas Weaver paused, took a drink of bottled water, and smiled. "That's probably enough of listening to me read, I think. Does anyone have any questions?"

The lady with the large bag, which had turned out to be her knitting raised her hand. "Yes. What happens to Timothy?"

Thomas laughed, and tapped the pile of books on the table. "That's what these are here for. They'll tell you exactly what happens to Timothy."

Dominick was tempted to raise his hand and say, "I've got a lot of questions," but he didn't. Instead, he waited until everyone else had run out of things to ask, doozies like: "Where do you get your ideas?" and "How much money did you get for writing it?" and "How much of this book really happened to you?"

Dominick was interested in that last question, but Thomas just said, "It's all fiction. Writers are paid to make things up, right?"

I call bullshit, Thomas. No way you could "make up" so many things that mirror what has happened to me.

Thomas made one last pitch—"I'll be happy to sign copies of the book for as long as you want to keep buying them tonight"—and the crowd gave him a polite round of applause. Several more people grabbed a copy and took it to the register to purchase it so they could get it signed.

Dominick wandered around the store, keeping an eye on Thomas, waiting for everyone else to disperse. It didn't take long. After ten minutes, Thomas had taken his sign down and was helping the clerk restock the copies that hadn't sold.

Dominick approached him and said, "Sorry, still got time to sign one more?"

"Of course!" Thomas said, and reached his hand out. "I suppose if I do a thousand of these, I'll get over the thrill of signing a book, but for now, it's still pretty cool."

As Thomas was signing the book, Dominick leaned over and said, "How many lives is this for you?"

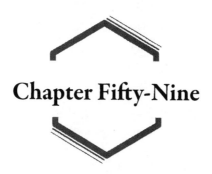

Chapter Fifty-Nine

The Sharpie Thomas was using to sign the book slipped, leaving a long dark trail across the dedication page. He sucked in his breath, and Dominick was surprised to see tears well in his eyes.

"Dude," Dominick said. "You would be a terrible poker player."

Thomas opened the book, flipped through the pages, then ran his finger down a few paragraphs. "I thought so. I didn't put that in the book. Someone else said that to me once." Thomas stared a long time at Dominick without saying anything.

He's trying to estimate the chances of whether that was a lucky guess, or if I'm going through the same thing he is.

"What are you doing tomorrow?" Thomas asked.

"Teaching school, just like every day."

"I've got a court appearance in the morning, but my late afternoon is free. Do you want to meet over at the batting cages by the Dairy Queen? Say, 4:30? We could hit a few balls around, and maybe talk a little."

"Yes, that sounds great. I think we've got a lot to talk about."

Thomas shook Dominick's hand, then under his breath and to himself, he said, "After all these years, you'd think I'd be ready for something like that ..."

BY THE TIME DOMINICK got to the batting cages the next day, Thomas was already there, looking very non-lawyerly in sweat pants and a ragged Middle Falls High School sweatshirt. Dominick watched him take a few swings. Thomas was never going to be a professional baseball player, that much was obvious. Where Zack was fluid and relaxed in everything he did, his brother seemed to have an extra motion where none was needed.

Thomas glanced over his shoulder and gave Dominick a nod. "Hope I don't intimidate you too much with my flailing away. This is where I come to work out my frustrations. This next ball is the judge that ruled against us this morning." He took a mighty swing, which missed the ball by half a foot.

"I hate it when the judge throws me a curveball like that."

Thomas waited another few seconds, but no more balls came. "Guess that's it. Your turn."

Dominick opened the cage and slipped past Thomas into the cage. He picked up one of the bats leaning against the backdrop, put two quarters into the machine, set it for "medium" and took his stance. He stood with his legs shoulder-width apart, hands a few inches up on the bat, the bat waving just a few inches off his shoulder.

Haven't swung at a baseball in twenty years, but it's like riding a bike, right?

The first ball came humming at him, belt high and over the outside corner. He swung, a graceful arc that wasn't even close to the ball.

Well, at least I didn't fall down. Damn, I'm getting old.

After a few more misses, he finally connected on a sizzling line drive to the back of the net.

Better.

By the end of his twenty balls, he was roping shots to all fields.

"I should have known," Thomas said from behind him. "You're like my damn brother—good at everything you touch."

"If you believe that, we should go bowling sometime. That will make you feel much better."

Thomas laughed and said, "Let's grab a Coke."

They went inside the snack bar that was attached to the cages, picked up a couple of sodas, and sat at the corner table, as far away from anyone as they could be. They leaned slightly forward, so their voices didn't need to carry.

"So. Same question. How many lives is this for you?"

Thomas was silent for two beats, then said, "Just my second. You?"

"Four. I'd like it to be my last, and go on to whatever's next, but I have this terrible fear that if I die of some terrible disease as a ninety year old man, I'm just going to wake up in the same place again."

Thomas nodded. "Yep. It's like we've been given this key piece of information—that there's something besides the void on the other side of death—but we still don't know much. And, what you and I are getting isn't anything like what any religion, prophet or guru ever foretold. I know this is a personal question, but did you suicide each time?"

"No. At the end of my first life, I tried to stop a boy from killing my students. He shot me, and I woke up as a nine year old."

"Nine? Damn, that's tough. I woke up as a fifteen year old, and that was tough enough. I can't imagine having to be a kid all over again. So," Thomas said, his logical mind working away, "you said, 'at the end of your first life?' What about the others?"

Dominick drew a deep breath. "Kind of hard to talk about with someone you just met. The last two times, I took my own life. Things weren't working out right, and I took the cowardly way out, hoping I could fix things if I had another chance."

"I understand. I nearly did the same. But then I met an old woman named Emily Leon, who told me to not lose hope. For some reason, I listened to her."

"Emily? That's funny. That's my wife's name." Dominick took a drink of his Coke, then said, "You know something? Even though neither one of us knows the answers, I feel better just finally having someone I can talk about this with. Sometimes, I think I'll go crazy from *not* talking about it, but there's too much risk."

Thomas nodded. "I've had two people I could talk about this with, my friend Carrie, and my mom."

"Are they both travelers, like us?"

"Carrie was. My mom, I actually convinced."

"I tried that once. It didn't go so well. That's how I ended up driving my car off an embankment at eighty miles an hour."

Thomas winced. "There's a lot of ways it can turn out bad."

"So, it feels like you're the only person I can talk to about this, but ..."

"Sure. Go ahead."

"My first life, I was killed by a student during a school shooting at Middle Falls. Yesterday, I saw that student again for the first time since that day. I have no idea what I'm going to do. Is he just going to march into my classroom and start shooting people again, any day now?"

"When did he do it in your first life?"

"December 1999."

"Fifteen months, then. We both know things don't turn out the same from life to life. Some things are better, some worse. But, for the most part, there is a symmetry between our repeating lives. I wouldn't think it would happen this early, but it's possible."

"So, what do I do, then?"

"You've got to be prepared."

Chapter Sixty

Over the next few months, Dominick did what he could to be better prepared.

He hung out with Thomas Weaver often—at least once a week. They were interested in a lot of the same things, and it was a major relief to know someone you could talk to about the one aspect of your life you couldn't talk about with anyone else. They even went bowling. Good as his word, Dominick was terrible, and Thomas beat him by thirty pins.

More often than not, they met at the batting cages, got a workout swinging at pitches, and then would hang out in the snack bar, swapping stories of what it was like to live multiple lives. Thomas asked if he could write Dominick's story, too.

"My book's selling pretty well, and the publisher is asking me if I've got a sequel in me. You're the only other time traveler I know. We could call it *The Death and Life of David Dellacroix*, or something like that. Pretty catchy, huh?"

"Thanks, but I don't feel the need to have my life fictionalized."

On the way out of the batting cages that day, they stopped and looked at the new bats hanging for sale on the wall. Thomas pulled one down, took its measure, then walked to the register and bought it.

He handed it to Dominick. "Here. Early birthday present. Or, late Christmas present. Whatever. Why don't you keep this somewhere in your classroom, just in case? Not that a bat does a lot of good against a gun, but you never know."

Dominick loved the bat, but thought he might need something with a little more punch, so he purchased several pistols, a .22 and a .45, and started hanging out at a shooting range on the south side of town.

If I'm going to have guns, I've got to make sure I know how to use them.

He had a hard time explaining his new interest in guns to Emily.

The day he brought them home, he put them both in a locked gun box in his closet, and stored the ammunition on a high shelf in the garage. Still, Emily didn't like it.

"I don't understand why you feel the need to arm yourself like that. Has something happened that you haven't told me about?"

Yes, but there's no way I can tell you. I hate lying to you more than anything except being separated.

"I just want to be able to protect us if need be."

"So, if a burglar breaks into the house in the middle of the night, you're going to unlock that box, grab the guns, then run out to the garage for bullets?"

"Would you rather I kept it loaded in my nightstand?"

Emily gave him *the look* which meant that was a question so stupid, it didn't need to be answered. And probably shouldn't have been asked.

Dominick hated sneaking around behind her back, but he did, to some extent. He waited until nights or weekends when she had something else to attend to before he went to the range and practiced. After a few months of not being confronted with the ongoing evidence, the whole issue faded into the background and was mostly forgotten.

Dominick also did his best to prepare for an attack by stopping it before it happened.

Over the course of Freshman English, Dominick gave extra time and attention to Gerald Fleischer. Early in the year, Dominick would flinch each time Gerald walked into the classroom, anticipating the worst. By the end of the semester, nothing untoward had happened. On the last day of class, he asked Gerald to stay behind for a moment.

He was a shorter boy who obviously gave very little thought or care to his appearance. His hair was normally greasy and slicked down, and up close he smelled oddly of slightly sour milk and old soup. He rarely made eye contact, and as he approached the desk, he said, "Did I do something wrong, Mr. Davidner?"

"No, not at all. It's been great having you in class this year. My wife and I have a house over on Periwinkle Street, and it needs painting. I was wondering if you'd be interested in helping me with it? I'm paying ten bucks an hour."

Dominick watched the wheels turn inside Gerald's brain. *God only knows what kind of things he's thinking about.*

"Are you going to be hiring anyone else to help?"

Ah. There we go. He's afraid that if anyone else shows up, he'll be low man on the totem pole again, and would probably end up getting bullied, to boot.

"No, just looking for one helper. I'm going to do most of the painting, but I need someone to help me tape everything off, fill my paint bucket, things like that. It won't be anything too tough."

Gerald narrowed his eyes, considering.

Come on, I'm trying to help you here.

"Okay, sounds good. I'll have to ask my parents, since they'll have to drive me. When are you starting?"

"Next Monday." Dominick jotted something on a piece of scrap paper. "Here's my phone number. Why don't you have your parents give me a call?"

THE NEXT MONDAY, GERALD'S mother pulled up to Dominick's house in an old four-door Plymouth. She got out with Gerald and walked toward Dominick, who was already outside, getting everything ready. She approached with an old brown purse clutched in front of her like a shield.

"Mr. Davidner?"

"Yes, how do you do?"

"I'm Mrs. Fleischer. Are you sure Gerald won't be any trouble?"

"Oh, no, not at all. He'll be a big help. He's always a hard worker in class."

Mrs. Fleischer's face twisted in a sour knot. Apparently, she did not agree with Dominick's assessment of her son's work ethic. "What time should I be back to pick him up?"

"Oh, we won't work too long today. We're just doing prep work. Maybe 2:00?"

She reached inside her purse, pulled out a wrinkled five dollar bill. "Here, this is in case you go out to lunch."

Dominick held up his hand. "No need, Mrs. Fleischer, my wife, Emily, is making us our lunch. She's a very good cook."

Lightning quick, the bill disappeared back in the purse. She turned to Gerald. "I'll be here at two." She turned and marched to the car and drove away.

Gerald risked a rare moment of eye contact to gauge Dominick's reaction to his mother.

Dominick smiled, slapped him on his shoulder, and said, "Well! She seems nice," and turned toward the paint supplies. He did not notice that Gerald moved away at his touch.

They spent the first hour laying everything out for the day, and talking. Dominick quizzed him about everything he could think of—what movies he liked, what books, what television shows. As it turned out, he never went to the movies, only read what he was assigned in school, and his parents only allowed him to watch PBS.

As they were taping the plastic over the windows, Dominick asked, "So, if you don't read, or watch television, what do you do with your time?"

"My parents own the pawn shop over on Halliday. I spend a lot of time helping out there."

Dominick snapped his fingers. *That's right. Fleischer Pawn. I'd never connected that before.*

"If I gave you a couple of books, would that be okay with your folks?"

"Maybe. What kind of books?"

This was the closest thing to actual interest in anything that Dominick had seen all day.

"Science fiction maybe?"

Gerald grinned. "That's probably close to the edge, but if it came from my English teacher, they'd probably let it go."

"Good enough. I'll grab a few from the house before you leave."

By the time they had all the windows covered, it was lunchtime. Emily had made her special tuna sandwiches and sliced up some watermelon. They ate at a picnic table in the backyard. Emily tried to draw Gerald out, but had even less success than Dominick had.

When lunch was over, Gerald asked if he could use their bathroom, and Dominick told him where it was in the house. When he disappeared inside, Emily laid her hand on Dominick's.

"Tough nut to crack, huh?"

"He doesn't fit in at school. I thought I'd take a chance and see if I could figure out what makes him tick."

I hate misleading you. As soon as I figure this out, I will never have to do it again.

By the time Mrs. Fleischer came by to pick up Gerald, they had two sides of the house prepped and ready for paint.

Before he left, Dominick went in the house and found his copies of *Glory Road* by Robert Heinlein, and *Fahrenheit 451* by Ray Bradbury. Two guaranteed winners, if he was willing to crack them open.

Dominick and Emily stood on the sidewalk in front of the house and waved at them as they pulled away. Neither of the Fleischers waved back.

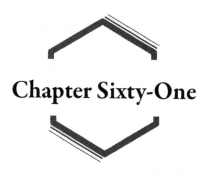

Chapter Sixty-One

The closer it drew to the date of his death in his first life, the more nervous and vigilant Dominick became. He even sewed a pocket inside his carrier bag that he took to school every day so that he could hide his .45 in there, where no one could see it.

Pretty sure that if I have to use it, the school district will frown on me bringing a loaded weapon to school, and I'll lose my job, and probably my whole career. But you know what? I'll still be alive. And, I'll still have Emily. I'll take it.

He didn't have Gerald in any classes that semester, but he made an effort to find him in the halls and at least say hello to him every day. He never seemed any more or less weird than he had all along.

The day finally arrived, and Dominick fought every instinct to call in sick and avoid the situation altogether.

Couldn't live with myself if I took that cowardly way out. What's the worst that could happen? I get shot and killed. I wake up as a nine year old again. And I have to wait eighteen years to see Emily again. Yeah, that's pretty bad.

Of course, they had already celebrated their anniversary in this life months earlier, so Emily attached no significance to the date at all. She rolled out of bed with an "oomph," got ready, and went off to school like she did every other day.

Dominick had considered buying a bulletproof vest to wear on this day, but remembered that he had been shot in the throat, and no vest would have saved his life. He got dressed in his normal clothes, but did make the allowance of wearing his sneakers instead of his oxfords, just in case he needed to move fast.

The day dragged by for Dominick. Every loud noise, every unexpected sound of any kind, made him jump. He looked for Gerald in the hallways between each class, but never saw him. Finally, he checked the absentee list to see his name was there. It wasn't. So he was somewhere in school, just invisible, apparently.

When sixth period finally arrived, he got to the classroom early. He unlocked the closet door and made sure everything was tidy inside, so he could move the kids there if need be. He briefly considered calling a safety drill and putting the whole class in the closet, but what was the play then? Keep them there all period long? It'd never work.

Many things were different from one life to the next. One of those was the book they were studying in this life. This time, it was *In Cold Blood* by Truman Capote, instead of *Lord of the Flies*.

Not sure that's a good omen.

It was AP English again, and so it was once again a small class, only seven students this time around. Dominick had prepared a lecture about how groundbreaking *In Cold Blood* had been, essentially inventing the genre of True Crime single-handedly, but when he stood at the front of the class to deliver it, he just wasn't in the mood. Instead, he had everyone move their desks into a circle, and he sat with them. He asked them what the book had made them feel, which parts had scared them, which parts had made them emotional.

He was surprised at the depth and variety of the responses. One girl said that she identified with the young girl who came to the Clutter house on that early morning, only to discover the horrific murder scene. "I don't know how she ever recovered from it," she said.

Doug, who had fallen under Gerald's aim in Dominick's first life, said that the offhand way the killer discussed the crime with the sheriff on the drive back to Kansas would stay with him. "How can you do something so horrible, and then be so casual about it?"

Dominick became engrossed in the conversation and jumped when the bell sounded, marking the end of the period. The kids in class laughed at him.

"You know, Mr. Davidner, that happens at the end of every class, right?" Doug asked.

"You know, Doug, I still haven't made out the grades for the semester, right?"

Doug's smile faded, but Dominick laughed and said, "Just kidding. I don't know where my head was at. Have a good weekend, everybody. We'll pick this up next week."

Just to be sure everything was copacetic, Dominick hustled over to the classroom door, opened it, and stuck his head outside before he let his class out. The hall was full of jostling, talking, rambunctious high school students, talking about a basketball game that was on tap for that evening in the gym.

At dinner that night, Emily said, "So what's been going on with you?"

"Who, me?" Dominick asked innocently.

"Yes, you. You've been so tightly wound the last few weeks, I thought you were going to snap and go postal on everyone."

Can't fool you, Em.

"Now, tonight, you seem your old self. So, what's up?"

There's no way for me to tell you, Emily. I can't tell you that tomorrow is the first day in more than forty years that will be completely new to me. I wish I could tell you how excited I am that there will finally be new movies for me to see, new books to read, new discoveries that I don't know about. Hell, for all I know, Microsoft stock will go in the tank next week, and there goes our nest egg. And I love it. Uncertainty is part of the flavor of life, and it's been missing for me for too many years. I can wake up tomorrow and have no idea what's coming.

"I'm sorry, Em. I wish I knew. Probably a combination of things, but I'm feeling better now. Hey, *The Green Mile* is playing at the Pickwick. Want to go see it this weekend?"

Emily wrinkled her nose. "Stephen King, right?"

"Yes, but, it's not a horror movie. Best of all, I've never seen it."

Emily laughed. "Well, of course you've never seen it. It just came out today, right?"

Dominick caught himself. "Right."

THE NEXT DAY, DOMINICK met Thomas at a coffee shop downtown. It was too cold to hit balls in the batting cage.

"Glad to see you're still in one piece," Thomas said, when he slid into the booth across from Dominick. "Happy emancipation day."

"I've never asked you this, but when does your emancipation day arrive? When do you finally get to start living new days?"

Thomas shook his head. "Not for a long time. I may not have been as young as you when I started over, but I traveled further back. I've got to get to 2016 before I start seeing anything completely new."

"I feel for you. I woke up today with a whole new attitude. Nothing like it. Hey, did I ever mention to you that I bought a few shares of Microsoft the day it IPOed?"

"No, but I did the same thing. What do you think put me through law school and bought my house? I never do this, but I'm just gonna tell you one thing. You might want to diversify your portfolio. It's not gonna exactly crash, but these are the glory days. You might want to look at Amazon."

"Amazon? Don't they keep losing money every quarter?"

"Yep, they lose money on every purchase, but they make it up in volume."

Dominick looked at Thomas funny.

"Sorry, that's an old car salesman joke. I'm not telling you what to do, but I'm moving out of Microsoft now and into Amazon. If you don't want the risk of doing that, you might just convert a good chunk of it to cash and put it in bonds. Last time around, there was something called a tech bubble that burst around 2001. Cash is not a bad position to be in. Besides, how rich do you need to be?"

Dominick thought of his little house, his life with Emily, his job that he loved, and the fact that he was once again breathing 'unbreathed' air in his life. "I think I'm already as rich as I need to be."

Chapter Sixty-Two

The year 2000 arrived amid threats of Y2K, but when midnight of January 1, 2000, swept across the planet, the planes stayed in the air, the banks kept functioning, and the world kept spinning on its axis.

As Thomas had suggested, Dominick diversified his portfolio. Ms. Jansen had left Tom Patterson's firm not long after the Microsoft IPO to open her own small brokerage. Dominick had used her until she retired in 1994, and he had been using her daughter, Janis, ever since.

On January 3rd, Dominick sold off ninety percent of his Microsoft stock, which felt like saying goodbye to an old friend. It did wonders for his liquidity, though. He purchased a few thousand shares of Amazon and swore to himself that he would let it sit and percolate, just as he had done with the Microsoft stock, no matter what happened over the next few years. The remaining cash, which was substantial, he put into bonds and did his best to forget about it.

When Dominick took stock of his life, he felt like he was coming up sevens across the board. It had been a long, strange trip to arrive back at this point, but he had accomplished what he had thought was impossible—he was even happier than he had been at the end of his first life.

THE DEATH AND LIFE OF DOMINICK DAVIDNER

IF YOU HAD ASKED HIM, Dominick would have told you that he hadn't relaxed that much in the weeks and months after his death anniversary. He would have told Thomas Weaver that he was still vigilant, watching around corners, always looking for danger.

Human nature is still human nature, though, and as time passed, his defenses lowered. It's impossible to stay on alert forever. The concept of *The Tyranny of Reality* says that we all tend to rely on the most recent information we have, especially if we've seen it with our own eyes. If you've watched your favorite baseball team win eleven games in a row, it's hard for the average fan to believe they won't win their twelfth. If you've dodged a date with a spree killer, it's easy to believe you'll keep on dodging it.

So it was for Dominick Davidner on Thursday, April 19, 2000.

He had kept the gun tucked away in its hidden pocket in his bag up until the Christmas break, but Dominick knew in his heart that a teacher carrying a gun to school was not good. So, over the holiday, he had taken the seam ripper, removed the pocket, and stored the gun back in its locked box on the top shelf of his closet.

He kissed Emily goodbye standing in their driveway, just as he did every day. He carefully told her, "I love you, Emily Davidner," just like he did every day. He drove the same route, got the same cup of coffee in the lounge. Everything about his day was happily, boringly normal, until sixth period.

The AP English Class had finished their reading of *In Cold Blood* and moved on to *To Kill a Mockingbird*. The seven students were reading the early chapters of the book. Dominick was grading their essay tests at the front of the class. Silence reigned, until Dominick heard the sound he had been listening for all year.

BANG! BANG! BANG!

Dominick's stomach fell and he experienced the strongest sense of déjà vu he'd ever had. He knew with absolute certainty that Gerald was coming to his room. The students all turned in their seats and looked around to see where the noise was coming from.

Dominick leaped up from the desk. He did his best to keep his voice calm, but adrenaline put a quiver into his words. "Hurry. Everyone. Get in the closet, now."

Most of the students sat, looking at him, absorbing his words. Michelle Landry jumped up, ran to the closet door and tugged on it. She turned back to Dominick. "It's locked."

Oh my God. What an idiot I am. I deserve to die for letting my guard down. These kids don't deserve anything, though.

He reached into his pocket, grabbed the keys and threw them to Doug, who snagged them one handed. "It's the steel key. Get that door unlocked and get in there. Now!"

Hearing the alarm in Dominick's voice spurred them all into action and they ran for the closet door. Dominick sprinted to the light switch and switched it off just as the door began to open. Dominick kicked the door as hard as he could. It slammed shut violently, and Dominick heard a meaty thud as the door connected with someone's face. He heard muffled swearing from the other side of the door.

Dominick groped behind him, looking desperately for something, but unable to take his eyes off the door. He glanced to his left and saw that Doug had opened the closet door and the last of the students scrambled inside, closing it behind them.

Better. Not perfect, but better.

One bullet, then another, ripped through the classroom door, shattering windows on the far side of the room. The door swung inward just as Dominick's hand closed on the smooth handle of the baseball bat he'd left leaning there.

Gerald Fleischer strode into the room, a Remington .30-06 rifle slung around his shoulder in place of the two handguns he had carried the previous lifetime.

Time slowed.

Gerald sensed movement to his left and turned his head and rifle in that direction.

Dominick launched himself forward. He swung the baseball bat with everything he had.

The rifle went off.

Chapter Sixty-Three

Carrie spun the pyxis clockwise, jumping it ahead days, months, and years. She touched it lightly, feathering it to a stop.

"This is a perfect example of what we're talking about. Watch."

She set time free, and it moved forward at normal speed.

An almost empty classroom showed on her pyxis. A man switched all the lights off, just as the door to the room opened. The man kicked it viciously and it slammed shut, hitting a boy carrying a rifle, and almost breaking his nose. The boy staggered back, shook his head, pointed the rifle and fired two shots into and through the door. The older man reached behind him and grabbed a weapon. The boy kicked the door open and stepped inside.

He saw movement to his left and raised the rifle, just as the man swung the bat.

The rifle fired first, and before the man could connect with the bat, he was shot in the throat. He spun around, dropped the bat, and fell to the floor.

"I watched something like this happen to this same man three lifetimes ago. I didn't do anything about it, because I didn't really know how, yet. He has lived three incomplete lives since then. Those lives have fed the Machine, but they have not been good for his psyche. It is deteriorating. Now I know what can be done."

Carrie reached inside the image, grabbed a fistful of it and pulled it toward her until it snapped. She rolled the material into a ball and dropped it into a hole in the floor.

"Now. Watch ... "

Chapter Sixty-Four

Dominick's bat connected with Gerald Fleischer's nose, spraying blood, blinding him.

Dominick leaped on top of Gerald, wrestled the rifle away from him and sent it skittering across the tile floor.

Dominick looked down and saw blood spreading across his blue shirt.

The bullet had ripped through Dominick's left side, and he felt himself grow dizzy, but he refused to get off Gerald, who was lying on his back, shaking his head violently from side to side.

"You broke my fuckin' nose!"

I'm gonna do worse than that to you right now.

Dominick raised the bat over his head to smash it down on his head, but strong hands grasped his wrist.

"Mr. Davidner. It's okay. I've got him," Doug said.

"I told you guys to stay in the closet! Watch him! He might have handguns on him."

Dominick's dizziness increased. His eyes rolled up in his head and he fell to his left.

Chapter Sixty-Five

When he opened his eyes again, he was on a gurney, being loaded onto an ambulance.

"Hold on, sir," the EMT said, putting an oxygen mask over his mouth and nose. We're taking you to the hospital."

From far away, Dominick heard Emily's voice.

"Nicky!" Her voice was a piercing scream of fright. He tried to lift up his head, but couldn't.

Then, there she was, her beautiful face a mask of fear.

"Nicky, Nicky, Nicky! What happened?"

"Ma'am, he really shouldn't try to speak right now. We're taking him to the hospital."

Dominick reached up with his hand and pushed the mask away. Emily leaned close so she could hear him. There were tears in his eyes, but he radiated relief.

"We made it, Em. We made it."

Chapter Sixty-Six

Carrie stood in front of the seven floating desks once again, but the environment felt very different than the last time she had been there. Then, she had been quaking, afraid that whatever these beings were, they might have the ability to scramble her soul to atoms and scatter them across the width of the universe.

Today, she didn't approach them as equals, because they obviously saw more of what actually Is than she did from her limited viewpoint. This time, however, they had sent a messenger—a small ball of floating light—to request her presence.

Carrie reached out and touched the ball of light and she was instantly transported before the council.

"Yes?" Carrie had asked.

"Thank you for being here," Blue-Robe said. "We were not properly introduced. My name is Harmonium."

"Pleased to meet you." *Yep, I can still manage a lie in front of the council. Good to know.* Carrie stared at Harmonium—the tilt of her head, the nervous fluttering of her hands inside the robe. *It's hard for me to believe, but it's almost like she's uncomfortable.*

"When you were here last, we had some unfinished business."

Do I get a raise, or is this just one of those jobs where you get a title instead?

"You were not the first person to be brought up on charges of interference. There was another before you. Her name was Emillion."

Wait. That's who Bertellia said Emily really was.

"The Council does not think it is right—"

Does the Council mean "fair?"

"—to have punished her for doing what is now our protocol. We'd like you to bring her back."

Chapter Sixty-Seven

Carrie walked along the nearly infinite row of desks. She stopped at each one, smiled, and laid a hand on the shoulder of each Watcher who occupied it. She talked with them about what they were seeing, the decisions they were making, and any problems they might have.

She came to an empty desk and sat down. She glanced to her left and saw that Margenta was seated beside her. "Oh, hello, Margenta. Blessings to you."

"Blessings," Margenta said, but the pleasantry cost her. She attempted to stop her lip from curling back in distaste, but failed. Her back ramrod straight, she manipulated her pyxis and did her best to ignore Carrie.

Carrie pulled out her pyxis and ran through her own charges. She had refused to give them up, even with her new responsibilities. No one knew the threads of their lives as she did.

She settled on Dominick Davidner and saw that he was sitting at his kitchen table, drinking coffee, talking and laughing with Emily-who-was-also-Emillion. His once-dark hair had broad streaks of gray in it and he had reading glasses perched on the end of his nose. Emily's hair had also begun to gray, but her peaceful, unlined face showed no signs of aging.

"Time for me to get to school," Emily said.

Dominick grabbed her waist and pulled her onto his lap. "How about we say this is your last year teaching? Thirty years at the same school should be enough and we sure don't need the money."

She kissed him sweetly. "I would love the time with you, but I would miss my kids." She stood and smoothed her sweater.

"I vote for the more time with me side of the equation, but you make up your own mind." He picked up his coffee cup and set it in the sink. "Oh, hey, I'm having lunch with Thomas this afternoon. It's a big day for him—an anniversary of some sort."

Carrie moved the scene back and played it again. She smiled at their happy life, and speaking only to herself, said, "They just said to bring her back. They didn't say *when*."

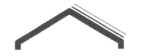

Available Now:
The Final Life of Nathaniel Moon[1]

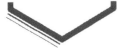

---

1. http://amzn.to/2z8seyk

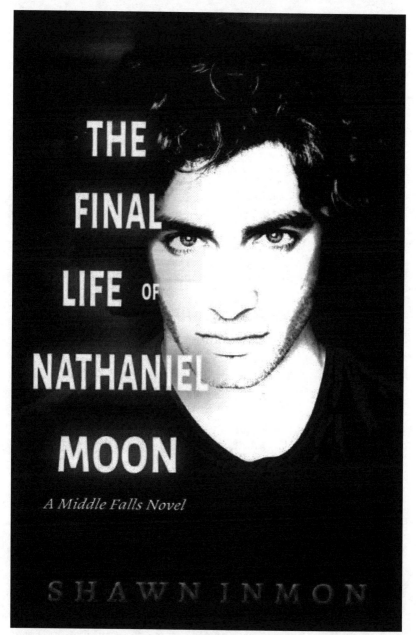

Author's Note

The Death and Life of Dominick Davidner was a much easier book for me to write than its predecessor in this series. I struggled mightily to get on track with *The Redemption of Michael Hollister*, and it showed –it took me almost a year to write, although I did manage three other books in the interim.

Dominick's story dropped into my head almost all at once, complete and ready to be written. I love it when that happens. Then, it feels more like I'm taking dictation, than actually creating something. In fact, I wrote it quickly—about 80% of the book was written between November 20th, and December 17th, 2017.

At its heart, I saw *Dominick* as a love story. Not a Romance, though – that has very definite tropes you need to hit, and I chose not to do that. Still, a love story, between Dominick and Emily.

When I introduced Emily as Emillion in *The Unusual Second Life of Thomas Weaver*, I saw her as a stand in for Clarence, the angel from *It's a Wonderful Life*. That's how I wrote her in that first book. But then, when she transitioned to human form, I saw her differently—a free spirit with her own unique view of the universe.

This book concludes the first trilogy in the *Middle Falls Time Travel* series. I think I managed to close all the circuits I had opened in the earlier books. We know, at least for the moment, how things turned out for Thomas (who finally got to his emancipation day at the very end of this story) Dominick, Emily, Michael, and Carrie.

There will be more books in the series, and the characters from these books will almost certainly pop up in them, as well, but it feels good to have the main characters' stories wrapped up here.

The fourth book in this series, *The Final Life of Nathaniel Moon*, will be out in March of 2018. It's the story I've had percolating in my brain the longest. In fact, I started writing it in 1980. Back then, I called it *The Man Who Is*. That terrible title sums up my writing ability at the time, and explains why it's taken me almost thirty-eight years to get back to it.

I've always been fascinated by how we, as a nation, can focus all our attention on one single story for a period of time. It doesn't matter if it's a baby down a well, a Long Island Lolita, or a missing Korean airplane—certain stories just grab the public consciousness. Often, when the cameras focuses on the key players in the drama, they turn out to be vapid people who have nothing to say, really. I've always wondered what would happen if someone who was at the center of one of those attention-grabbing events actually had something worthwhile to say. *The Final Life of Nathaniel Moon* will show what my answer to that is.

Writing a book is a lonely business—long hours sitting alone at the keyboard, trying to catch up to the story in your mind. Producing a book is a team effort, though, and I am so fortunate to have these people on my team:

Linda Boulanger from Tell Tale Book Covers designed the cover, and I love it. Linda and I have been working together since I first dipped my toe into publishing in 2012. There are times that we struggle to find the right concept. My *Lap Around America* book must have gone through close to a dozen iterations before we struck a winner. Not so with this book though. The cover you see is very close to the first one Linda sent me. To tell you how much I love working with her, she's already designed the cover for the next book in the series, too.

This marks the first book I have worked with Dan Hilton as my editor, but it won't be the last. He worked not only hard, but quickly and with a deft touch, untangling my sometimes-tangled sentences, and fixing my grammar, which I am the first to admit, is not what it could be. I appreciate everything he did to make this book a better experience for you.

Debra Galvan and Mark Sturgill acted as my proofreaders again. Debra has been with me for years now, and I trust her to not only find and eradicate whatever typos I make, but to make comments that always leave me chuckling. Mark hasn't been with me as long, but I have grown to trust his eye for details. When he tells me I need to check something, I always know I need to check it.

The talented writer Terry Schott, who is my writing BFF, was once again my alpha reader, which means he sees the truly rough first draft and makes gentle suggestions as to what might make a better story. Even more importantly, when my spirits flag, he is always there to pick me up and give me encouragement to go on. He's the man.

My bride, Dawn Adele, sits beside me as I write and puts up with my endless questions when something evades my mind. She is also a brilliant story creator, who has unerring instincts as to what works and what doesn't in a story. Many of the tasty bits of this book came directly from her.

I have a wonderful group of beta readers, as well, including Laura Heilman, Jeff Hunter, Joni Furry, Athena Herder, Carmen Anslow, Barb Larson, Marta Rubin, Dale Lewis, Kerri Lookabaugh, Craig Simmons (who got name-checked as a smokejumper in this book), and Kianne Werrell. They suffer through early drafts, so you don't have to.

I have at least three more *Middle Falls* books planned for 2018. I hope to see you between the pages of one of them soon.

Shawn Inmon
Seaview WA

December 2017

Made in the USA
Monee, IL
28 August 2024

64708739R00171